# Respiration

**International Review of Thoracic Diseases**

Founded 1944 as 'Schweizerische Zeitschrift für Tuberkulose und Pneumonologie' by E. Bachmann, M. Gilbert, F. Häberlin, W. Löffler, P. Steiner and E. Uehlinger, continued 1962–1967 as 'Medicina Thoracalis'



KARGER

Printed in Switzerland
on acid-free paper by
Thür AG Offsetdruck, Pratteln

Appears bimonthly:
1 volume per year (6 issues)

Respiration

**Submission:** Original papers written in English, German or French will be considered but articles in English are preferred. They should be sent to:

S. Karger AG
Editorial Dept. 'Respiration'
P.O. Box
CH-4009 Basel (Switzerland)

Manuscripts should be submitted in triplicate (with three sets of illustrations of which one is an original), typewritten double-spaced on one side of the paper, with a wide margin.

**Conditions:** All manuscripts are subject to editorial review. Manuscripts are received with the explicit understanding that they are not under simultaneous consideration by any other publication. Submission of an article for publication implies the transfer of the copyright from the author to the publisher upon acceptance. Accepted papers become the permanent property of 'Respiration' and may not be reproduced by any means, in whole or in part, without the written consent of the publisher. It is the author's responsibility to obtain permission to reproduce illustrations, tables, etc. from other publications.

**Arrangement**

*Title page:* The first page of each paper should indicate the title (main title underlined), the authors' names, and the institute where the work was conducted. A short title for use as running head and a translation of the complete title into English as well as the full address of the author to whom correspondence should be sent are also required.

*Full address:* The exact postal address complete with postal code must be given at the bottom of the title page. Please also supply Phone, Fax, and E-mail numbers.

*Key words:* For indexing purposes, a list of 3–10 key words in English is essential.

*Abstract:* Each paper needs an abstract of up to 10 lines in English and a summary of not more than 20 lines in the original language.

*Small type:* Paragraphs which can or must be set in smaller type (case histories, test methods, etc.) should be indicated with a 'p' (petit) in the margin on the left-hand side.

*Footnotes:* Avoid footnotes. When essential, they are numbered consecutively and typed at the foot of the appropriate page.

*Tables and illustrations:* Tables and illustrations (both numbered in Arabic numerals) should be prepared on separate sheets. Tables require a heading and figures a legend, also prepared on a separate sheet. For the reproduction of illustrations, only good drawings and original photographs can be accepted; negatives or photocopies cannot be used. When possible, group several illustrations on one block for reproduction (max. size 181 × 223 mm) or provide crop marks. On the back of each illustration, indicate its number, the author's name, and 'top'.

*Color illustrations:* Up to 6 color illustrations per page can now be integrated with the text at the reduced price of SFr. 600.–/US$ 400.00 per page. Color illustrations are reproduced at the author's expense.

*References:* In the text identify references by Arabic numerals [in square brackets]. Material submitted for publication but not yet accepted should be noted as 'unpublished data' and not be included in the reference list. The list of references should include only those publications which are cited in the text. Do not alphabetize; number references in the order in which they are first mentioned in the text. The surnames of the authors followed by initials should be given. There should be no punctuation other than a comma to separate the authors. Cite all authors, 'et al' is not sufficient. Abbreviate journal names according to the Index Medicus system. (Also see International Committee of Medical Journal Editors: Uniform requirements for manuscripts submitted to biomedical journals. Br Med J 1988; 296:401–405.)

*Examples*

*(a) Papers published in periodicals:* Kauffman HF, van der Heide S, Beaumont F, Blok H, de Vries K: Class-specific antibody determination against *Aspergillus fumigatus* by means of the enzyme-linked immunosorbent assay. III. Comparative study: IgG, IgA, IgM ELISA titers, precipitating antibodies and IgE binding after fractionation of the antigen. Int Arch Allergy Appl Immunol 1986;80:300–306.

*(b) Monographs:* Matthews DE, Farewell VT: Using and Understanding Medical Statistics. Basel, Karger, 1985.

*(c) Edited books:* Hardy WD Jr, Essex M: FeLV-induced feline acquired immune deficiency syndrome: A model for human AIDS; in Klein E (ed): Acquired Immunodeficiency Syndrome. Prog Allergy. Basel, Karger, 1986, vol 37, pp 353–376.

*SI-Units:* Since the United States of America and other countries outside Europe where 'Respiration' is read, have not accepted the SI-System, authors using SI-Units should add the conventional units in brackets, for example: $pO_2$ = 10 kPa (75 mm Hg).

*Further details:* Authors may consult our leaflet 'Rules for the Preparation of Manuscripts', available on request from the Publisher, S. Karger AG, P.O. Box, CH-4009 Basel (Switzerland).

**Page charges:** There is no page charge for papers of 4 or fewer printed pages (including tables, illustrations and references). Each additional complete or partial page is charged to the author at SFr. 245.– / US$ 196.00. The allotted size of a paper is equal to approx. 12 manuscript pages (including tables, illustrations and references).

**Galley proofs:** Unless indicated otherwise, galley proofs are sent to the first-named author and should be returned with the least possible delay. Alterations made in galley proofs, other than the correction of printer's errors, are charged to the author. No page proofs are supplied.

**Reprints:** Order forms and a price list are sent with the galley proofs. Orders submitted after the issue is printed are subject to considerably higher prices. Allow five weeks from date of publication for delivery of reprints.

KARGER

Respiration

**Publication data:** 'Respiration' is published 6 times annually. Volume 62 with 6 issues appears in 1995.

**Subscription rates:** Subscriptions run for a full calendar year. Prices are given per volume.

*Personal subscription:*

*Subscription + postage and handling*
SFr. 399.70 + SFr. 17.90 Europe
SFr. 399.70 + SFr. 27.30 Overseas
US$ 307.30 + US$ 17.90
(Must be in the name of, billed to, and paid by an individual. Order must be marked 'personal subscription'.)

*Institutional subscription:*

*Subscription + postage and handling*
SFr. 571.– + SFr. 25.50 Europe
SFr. 571.– + SFr. 39.– Overseas
US$ 439.00 + US$ 25.50

Airmail postage: SFr. 36.–, US$ 30.00. (Extra per volume.)

*Discount subscription prices:*
European Society of Pneumology

**Microforms:** Please direct all enquiries and orders to:
University Microfilms Inc.
300 North Zeeb Road, P.O. Box 1346
Ann Arbor, MI 48106-1346 (USA)

**Subscription orders:** Orders can be placed at agencies, bookstores, directly with the Publisher S. Karger AG, P.O. Box, CH-4009 Basel (Switzerland) or with any of the following distributors:

*Deutschland:* S. Karger GmbH, Postfach
D-79095 Freiburg

*France:* Librairie Luginbühl
36, bd de Latour-Maubourg, F-75007 Paris

*Great Britain, Ireland:* S. Karger Publishers
11 Ravenscroft Road
Beckenham, Kent BR3 4TP

*USA:* S. Karger Publishers, Inc.
26 West Avon Road, P.O. Box 529
Farmington, CT 06085

*India, Bangladesh, Sri Lanka:*
S. Karger India Subscription Agency
B-5/132 Safdarjung Enclave
New Delhi-110029

*Japan:* Katakura Libri, Inc.
36-9 Hongo 3-chome, Bunkyo-ku, Tokyo 113

**Change of address:** Both old and new address should be sent to the subscription source.

**Single issues and back volumes:** Information can be obtained through the Publisher.

**Advertising:** Correspondence and rate requests should be addressed to the Publisher.

**Bibliographic indices:** This journal is regularly listed in bibliographic services, including *Current Contents®*.

**Book Reviews:** Books are accepted for review by special agreement.



KARGER

# Inhalation Therapy

Roche and Genentech Symposium

European Cystic Fibrosis Conference
June 1–3, 1994, Paris, France

Guest Editors
*Ch. Koch,* Copenhagen, Denmark
*E. Puchelle,* Reims, France

16 figures, 5 tables, 1995

KARGER

**Respiration**

Vol. 62, Supplement 1, 1995

S. Karger
Medical and Scientific Publishers
Basel · Freiburg · Paris · London
New York · New Delhi · Bangkok
Singapore · Tokyo · Sydney

Drug Dosage
The authors and the publisher have exerted every effort to ensure that drug selection and dosage set forth in this text are in accord with current recommendations and practice at the time of publication. However, in view of ongoing research, changes in government regulations, and the constant flow of information relating to drug therapy and drug reactions, the reader is urged to check the package insert for each drug for any change in indications and dosage and for added warnings and precautions. This is particularly important when the recommended agent is a new and/or infrequently employed drug.


Printed in Switzerland on acid-free paper by
Thür AG Offsetdruck, Pratteln
ISBN 3-8055-6164-4

# Contents

Respiration 1995;62(suppl 1):1

*C. Koch*

National University Hospital,
Rigshospitalet, Copenhagen, Denmark

# Introduction

Respiratory complications, arising from acute and chronic infections leading to inflammation, retention of large quantities of viscous mucus, and tissue damage, are the major cause of morbidity and mortality in cystic fibrosis (CF). Accordingly, many CF treatments are targeted at the respiratory disease. Aimed at providing optimal therapeutic benefit, such medications are often delivered by inhalation. The perceived advantages are that drugs in an aerosol formulation will be delivered more efficiently to the site of infection in the respiratory tract, enabling lower doses to be administered, and with reduced potential for systemic absorption and toxicity.

This supplement to *Respiration* contains the proceedings of the plenary symposium 'Inhaled Therapy' held recently in Paris, France, during the 19th European Cystic Fibrosis Conference (ECFC). A panel of international speakers offered current perspectives on the pathophysiological processes underlying CF pulmonary disease, the effectiveness of well-established and novel inhalation therapies, and various factors which may compromise efficient delivery of such treatments.

The altered properties of airway secretions that contribute to respiratory disease in CF are reviewed by Dr. E. Puchelle (Reims, France) who also considers new pharmacological approaches aimed at restoring or improving mucociliary and cough transport. The underlying pathology of CF respiratory disease is further discussed by Dr. P. Birrer (Berne, Switzerland) in terms of the damaging effects of proteases in CF airway inflammation and proposed therapeutic strategies involving the administration of antiproteases such as $\alpha_1$-antitrypsin.

Dr. F. Faurisson (Paris, France) highlights the importance of nebulizer selection and performance, reviewing a recent study conducted by the Nebulizer Study Group of the French Cystic Fibrosis Association which demonstrates that optimal aerosol delivery is dependent upon a variety of factors including the drug/nebulizer combination used. Differences in nebulizer devices are also considered by Professor A. Smith (Seattle, Wash., USA) in an overview of aerosol antibiotic therapy; antibiotics have been administered for over 50 years and Professor Smith discusses a number of clinical studies with many different antibiotic agents. The issue of benefit to the patient is still somewhat controversial and may be related to differences in study design leading to inconsistent results. However, several studies with β-lactams, polymyxins and aminoglycosides have clearly demonstrated the clinical benefits of inhalation antibiotic therapy. Development of resistance and colonization with intrinsically resistant species of organisms are examples of potential hazards of prolonged treatment with inhalation antibiotics.

Recently, much interest has been generated by the approval of the novel enzymatic agent, recombinant human deoxyribonuclease (rhDNase or Dornase alfa pINN) for CF treatment in various European countries, the USA and elsewhere. Dr. M. Hodson (London, UK) provides an update on the major clinical studies involving rhDNase, particularly follow-up data on long-term treatment in mildly to moderately ill CF patients and the results of an open-label study of severely ill patients. Administered as an aerosol formulation, rhDNase has been demonstrated to significantly improve pulmonary function, and also to reduce the risk of clinical exacerbations of the lung disease.

Continuing advances in our understanding of the underlying processes of CF respiratory disease, the development of effective inhalation therapies such as rhDNase, and increasing awareness of factors which may influence optimal drug delivery, together provide an optimistic outlook for the management of CF. Although the genetic and clinical complexity of the disease means that there is still much to be clarified, it appears that there is every reason to believe that the future for CF patients is brighter than ever before.

Respiration 1995;62(suppl 1):2–12

E. Puchelle
S. de Bentzmann
J.M. Zahm

INSERM U 314, CHR Maison-Blanche, Reims, France

# Physical and Functional Properties of Airway Secretions in Cystic Fibrosis – Therapeutic Approaches

**Key Words**
Airway secretions
Cystic fibrosis
Lubrication
Mucolytics
Mucus rheology
Mucus transport

**Abstract**
The airway secretions which line the respiratory tract form a biphasic layer composed of an aqueous 'sol' layer and a more superficial 'gel' layer. In the sol layer, also described as the 'periciliary' layer or 'airway surface fluid', the cilia beat and relax. The lubricant sol layer enables the gel mucus present at the tips of the cilia to be transported by the ciliary beating of the ciliated cells. Due to difficulties with sampling, little is known about the physical and biochemical properties of the sol layer. The gel layer is composed of high molecular weight glycoproteins (mucins) linked with proteins and lipids. They form a gel network with a high water content (95%) and rheologic and physical properties (viscoelasticity, adhesivity) adapted in normal conditions to protect the airway mucosa, particularly through mucociliary transport. The adhesive properties of mucus, which are influenced by its lipid composition and degree of hydration, are very important in controlling the efficacy of mucus transport through ciliary activity and coughing. An intermediate viscosity and elasticity is required for optimal mucociliary transport. In obstructive airway diseases, either of genetic origin, such as cystic fibrosis (CF), or acquired (acute or chronic bronchitis), and particularly during inflammatory and infectious episodes, mucus dehydration is associated with an increase in secreted or transudated molecules and with marked augmentation of DNA content. These abnormalities contribute to the increased viscosity and adhesivity of the airway secretions and are responsible for their abnormally low transport rate by ciliary activity and for inefficient cough clearance. In view of these alterations in the physical and functional properties of CF airway secretions, pharmacologic approaches should aim to rehydrate the mucus and to restore normal mucociliary or cough transport by stimulating chloride ion secretion (i.e. using UTP or ATP associated with amiloride in order to block sodium ion and water reabsorption). During acute episodes of infection, recombinant human DNase (rhDNase) may rapidly prevent mucus stasis by improving its rheologic properties. Lubrication of the mucus at the sol phase interface by 'surfactant' therapy may also represent a very promising therapeutic perspective to reduce the hyperviscosity and hyperadhesivity of airway secretions.

## Introduction

In healthy subjects, the secretions which line the respiratory tract form an efficient barrier against exogenous particles; they entrap bacteria and noxious agents and transport them out of the airways by means of ciliary beating. Indeed, the mucus secreted by the surface and glandular airway cells has several fundamental protective functions involving mucociliary transport, humidification, waterproofing, insulation and antibacterial activity.

The mucociliary epithelium lining the airways forms a biphasic layer composed of an aqueous 'sol' layer (7–10 μm), known as the 'periciliary' layer or 'airway surface fluid' (ASF), in which the cilia beat and relax, and a more

Dr. E. Puchelle
INSERM U 314, CHR Maison-Blanche
45, rue Cognacq-Jay
F–51092 Reims Cedex (France)


0025–7931/95/0627–0002
$8.00/0

superficial 'gel' layer (0.5–2 μm) which lies over the tips of the cilia. The sol layer acts as a lubricant assisting the coordinated movement of the cilia which transport the gel layer and its aerocontaminants.

The sol layer is a permanent source of water in the airways. It can be used to replace the volume lost due to mucus swelling during exocytosis and thus maintain an optimal thickness of the sol layer surrounding the cilia. Mucus exocytosis and ion-water secretions are thought to occur concomitantly via intracellular calcium concentration changes.

**Table 1.** Chemical composition (%) of airway secretions from patients with laryngectomy, bronchiectasis and cystic fibrosis

| | Laryngectomy | Bronchiectasis | Cystic fibrosis |
|---|---|---|---|
| Water | 94.8 ± 1.9 | 94.8 ± 1.1 | 89.4 ± 2.2 |
| Protein | 1.0 ± 0.3 | 2.04 ± 0.4 | 5.6 ± 2.0 |
| Carbohydrate | 0.9 ± 0.2 | 1.05 ± 0.1 | 1.1 ± 0.2 |
| Lipid | 0.8 ± 0.3 | 1.2 ± 0.4 | 3.1 ± 0.9 |
| DNA | 0.02 | 0.08 | 0.41 |

Data obtained from references 2 and 4.

## Normal Airway Secretions

*Biochemical Properties*

Due to difficulties with sampling, little is known about the biochemical composition and rheologic properties of 'normal' airway secretions. Most of our knowledge on the normal composition of airway secretions originates from samples of sputum collected following inhalation of aerosolized hypertonic saline, the application of irritants such as citric acid or diverse mucus inducers such as prostaglandins, acetylcholine or histamine [1]. Whatever the collection method chosen, the quantity of mucus available for biochemical and rheologic analyses is very limited. Collecting airway secretions from laryngectomized or intubated subjects may appear an interesting approach [2, 3], however, it is possible that stimulated mucus differs from native mucus. In fact, most information on the composition of mucus is obtained from expectorated human airway secretions. According to Matthews et al. [2], Potter et al. [4] and Boat et al. [5], airway secretions consist of approximately 95% water and 5% solids. The solid component consists of about 2–3% proteins and glycoproteins, 1% lipids and 1% minerals. It has previously been reported that airway secretions from tracheotomized and laryngectomized patients are hypertonic compared with plasma. This hypertonicity most probably results from evaporation on the airway surface following inhalation of non humidified air. Recent results from Joris et al. [6], using ultramicroanalytic techniques to analyze ASF microsamples collected from human airways in vivo, have shown that 'normal' ASF is hypo-osmolar (about 220 mosm). They suggest that sodium reabsorption (in excess of water) is largely responsible for the regulation of the final ASF volume as sodium absorption appears to be the predominant transport component in unstimulated native epithelial tissue.

Mucus glycoproteins (or mucins) secreted by the goblet cells of the epithelium and by the mucous glands of the respiratory mucosa represent the major biochemical component of airway secretions [7]. These mucins are high molecular weight (HMW) polydisperse glycoproteins consisting of approximately 80% carbohydrate which is linked to a peptide backbone with sialic acid and sulfate on the carbohydrate side chains. There is increasing evidence that the diversity of these side chains allows the recognition and adhesion of bacteria which, in turn, maintain the sterility of the respiratory tract. Proteoglycans are also reported to be secreted from epithelial cells. Among these, hyaluronic acid, chondroitin sulphate and dermatan sulphate have been detected in airway secretions of smokers, asthmatics and CF patients [5, 8, 9]. HMW glycoproteins, such as mucins and proteoglycans, are important determinants of the rheologic properties of mucus. They are both thought to contribute to the surface properties of the mucus/airway epithelium interface which, in turn, determines the degree of lubrication at the surface of the respiratory epithelium [10].

Several glycoproteins, other than mucins, are directly involved in the airway mucosa antibacterial defence. These include secretory IgA (S-IgA), IgG, lysozyme and lactoferrin [11]. Peroxidase has also been identified in the secretory cells and glands of the surface epithelium and appears to possess activity against bacteria, viruses and mycoplasma. The anti-protease activity of airway secretions is mediated primarily by secretory leukoprotease inhibitor (SLPI) – a cationic protein found in serous secretory glandular cells.

All of these biochemical components directly contribute to the rheologic and physical properties of airway secretions (table 1, fig. 1). Glycoprotein-protein and pro-

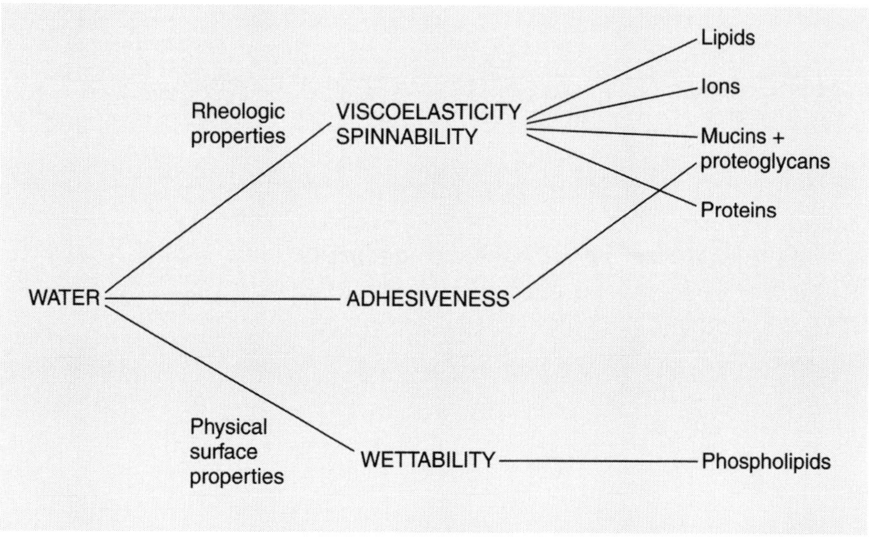


**Fig. 1.** Relationships between physical and biochemical properties of respiratory mucus.

teoglycan-protein interactions play a major role in determining the gel properties of airway secretions. Significant correlations have also been reported between mucin content, secretory proteins such as S-IgA and lysozyme, and viscoelasticity. Similarly, mucin-lipid interactions are likely to determine the surface-active properties of mucus. The water content, ionic concentration and pH of airway secretions may alter the rheologic properties by interfering with the degree of cross-linking of macromolecules. The negatively charged mucins (sulphated and carboxylic mucins) may also interact with positively charged proteins (lysozyme, SLPI) or cations such as calcium and magnesium via electrostatic bonds. Although a limited number of studies have investigated the lipid composition of airway secretions, it is now well established that phospholipids are present in the serous and mucous secretory granules of the submucosal glands and that they are released into the airway lumen or adsorbed onto the glycocalyx of the surface epithelial cells [12]. This epithelial coating of phospholipids and mucin-like molecules may act as a lubricant surface in mucus transport in addition to playing a protective role against the noxious pericellular environment [13]. Lipid-glycoprotein and lipid-protein crosslinks are strong interactions which are important in the control of the viscoelastic properties of mucus [14].

*Physical and Rheologic Properties*

Respiratory mucus is a very complex biologic material which possesses both flow and deformation (viscoelastic) properties characterized by non-linear (non-Newtonian

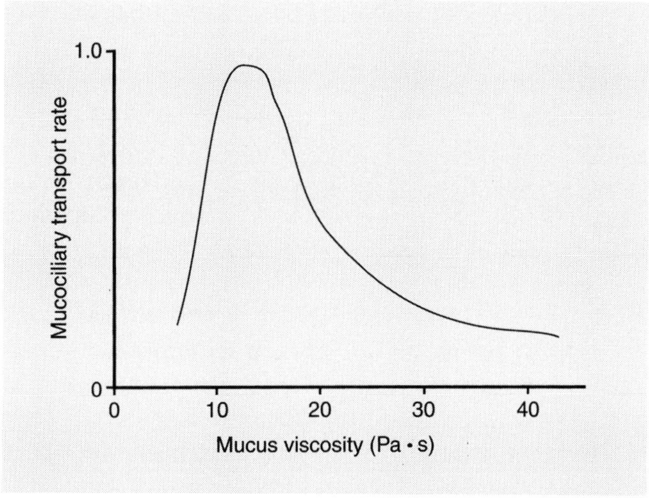


**Fig. 2.** Typical relationship between mucus viscosity and mucociliary transport rate. A low viscosity (<5 Pa·s) or a high viscosity (>20 Pa·s) results in inefficient mucociliary transport activity.

viscosity) and time-dependent behaviour (thixotropy). It also possesses surface properties, such as adhesiveness and wettability. These latter physical characteristics, which are independent of the viscoelastic properties, determine the capacity of mucus to protect, hydrate and lubricate the underlying airway epithelium and, therefore, are probably at least as important as the rheologic properties.

*Viscoelasticity.* Mucus is a highly non-Newtonian viscoelastic material. Under a discontinuous stress, induced

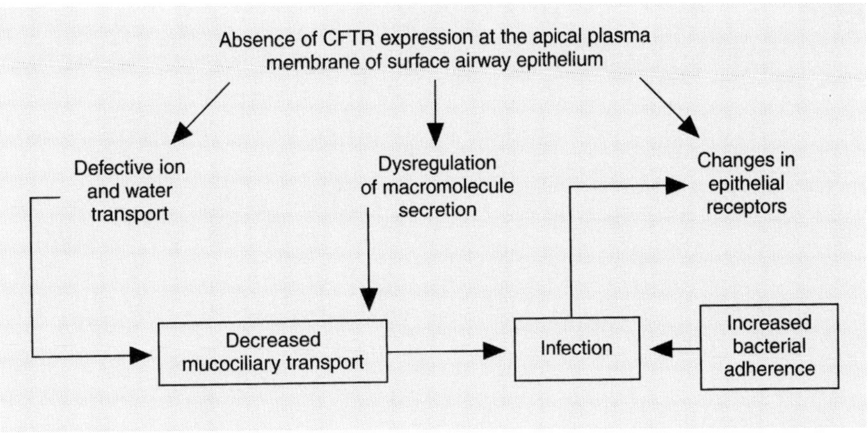


**Fig. 3.** Absence of or limited CFTR expression at the apical plasma membrane of the CF surface airway epithelium induces functional abnormalities in secretions of ions, water and macromolecules, resulting in decreased mucociliary transport and progressive purulent secretions with chronic infection usually by *P. aeruginosa*.

by ciliary motion during active ciliary beating or by coughing, the mucus instantaneously deforms. Once the stress is removed the mucus relaxes. Using standardized preparations of biopolymers to simulate normal and pathologic respiratory mucus, we were able to demonstrate that intermediate viscosity of about 15 Pa·s measured at a shear rate of 0.1 $s^{-1}$ represents an optimal rheologic profile for mucus transport. A low or a very high viscosity is inefficient for mucus transport (fig. 2).

*Wettability and Adhesiveness.* These two properties contribute markedly to the optimal interface characteristics between airway secretions and the surface epithelium, and between the sol and gel phases of mucus. These properties, which can be analyzed in terms of work of adhesion [14], therefore directly contribute to the efficiency of ciliary and cough clearance.

*Spinnability.* This is a property common to most types of mucus and is characterized by the ability of the mucus to be drawn into long threads under a 'tractor' effect. There is no close correlation between viscosity, elasticity and spinnability (the latter index providing information on the internal cohesion forces of mucus). However, the mucociliary transport rate correlates significantly with spinnability [15].

*Mucus Transport*

In healthy subjects, the mucociliary system provides a unique mechanism by which the respiratory epithelium may be cleared and the respiratory tract kept sterile.

The mucus gel layer acts as a coupler which transfers momentum from the tips of the cilia to the gel. In normal airways, the loads trapped by the gel mucus are transported by ciliary beating up to the esophagus where they are swallowed. The efficiency of mucociliary transport depends on several factors, including the number and activity of the cilia, the thickness of the sol and upper gel layer of mucus as well as their respective rheologic properties [16]. In healthy subjects, it has been demonstrated that a large variation in nasal mucus transport may occur in different subjects. This is related to the rheologic properties of the mucus and not to ciliary activity [17].

The viscoelasticity of mucus is one of the primary determinants of mucociliary clearance. From reports in the literature [18], it appears that decreasing mucus elasticity or viscosity enhances mucociliary transport. However, it has also been demonstrated that a further decrease in mucus elasticity results in a decreased mucus transport rate [19]. Our results support the concept that mucociliary transport reaches a peak and then decreases as viscosity is increased further [20].

## Pathologic CF Airway Secretions

Cystic fibrosis (CF) is a chronic hereditary disease characterized by an excessive production of airway secretions which results in bronchial obstruction and recurrent episodes of respiratory tract infections. Due to mutation of the cystic fibrosis transmembrane conductance regulator (CFTR) and particularly the mislocation or absence of CFTR expression at the apical plasma membrane of surface airway epithelium [21], several major abnormalities are observed: defective chloride secretion and increased sodium absorption result in decreased water secretion and an increase in the reabsorption of periciliary fluid. This, in turn, results in dehydration of the secretions and decreased mucociliary transport (fig. 3). The abnormal localization of CFTR in the ciliated cells and secretory

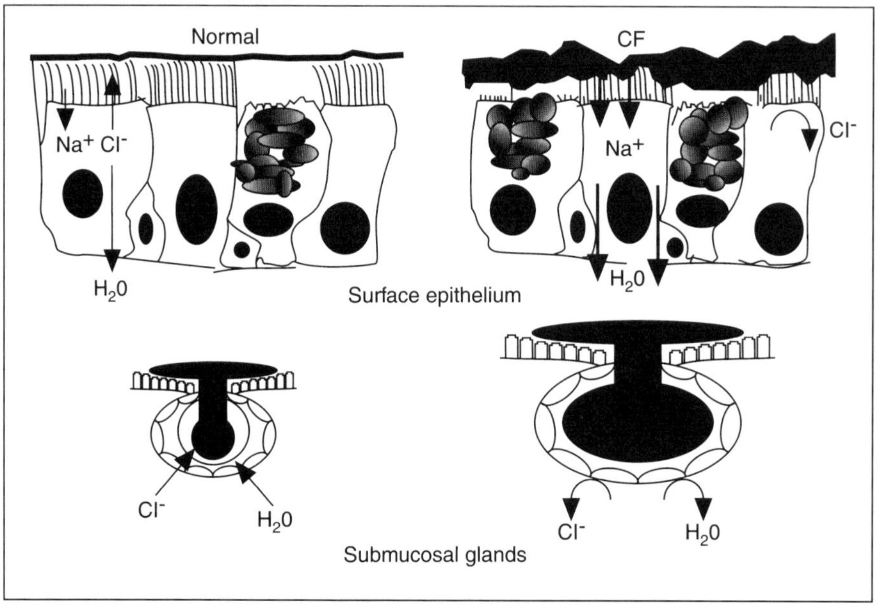


**Fig. 4.** A defective regulation of secretory chloride channels related to CFTR mutation and increased sodium absorption are identified at the airway surface epithelium and result in mucus dehydration with loss of mucociliary transport and submucosal gland enlargement.

granule membranes [22, 23] is thought to be responsible for the inability of the mucins packed inside the secretory granules to swell and pass from the 'condensed' phase (inside the granules) to the 'expanded' gel phase. If mucin expansion does not occur, mucus remains anchored to the surface of the airway epithelium, preventing mucus gel formation and therefore efficient mucociliary transport (fig. 4). In CF, dysregulation of macromolecule secretion, due to a defective acidification of the intracellular organelles (secondary to the loss of active chloride channels) induces a defective terminal glycosylation which results in a marked alteration of the sialylation of glycolipids. It is well established that CF airway secretions differ significantly from normal secretions in their water content and chemical composition compared with those of laryngectomy and bronchiectasis patients (table 1). In addition, there is a marked increase in protein and lipid content, while DNA content is increased 20-fold compared with that of laryngectomy and bronchiectasis mucus. This is of major importance since augmentation of DNA concentration is known to be directly associated with an increase in mucus viscosity [4, 5].

It has been reported that lipids, and particularly total phospholipids, are increased in CF compared with normal airway secretions [24, 25]. Moreover, Girod et al. [25] have demonstrated that in CF airway secretions, rigidifying fractions of phospholipids such as sphingomyelin, phosphatidylinositol and phosphatidylserine predominate to the detriment of surface-active fractions such as phosphatidylcholine and phosphatidylglycerol. This shift in phospholipid profile induces changes in the viscoelasticity as well as the surface properties of CF airway secretions. Together with mucus dehydration and hyperviscosity, this phospholipid imbalance may induce alterations in surface properties (augmentation of mucus adhesivity and stickiness) which are, in turn, responsible for impairment of mucus transport and severe bronchial obstruction. In other words, a high content of rigidifying fractions and a low content of surface-active fractions result in a high energy requirement to separate mucus from the surface mucosa. This increased work of adhesion is thought to be responsible for the inefficient clearance of mucus in CF.

Purulent sputum samples with a low water content are characterized by high values of adhesivity (the degree of adhesivity corresponds with the force which must be applied to separate the adhesive fluid [mucus] from the adherent surface [the airway mucosa] in vivo). Figure 5 highlights this close correlation between water content (expressed as dry weight) and adhesive properties of CF mucus. The lower the water content, the higher the adhesivity and the lower the mucus transport rate by ciliary activity [10].

Although cough does not contribute to airway clearance in healthy subjects, it may account for more than 50% of clearance in patients with hypersecretion, compensating for defective mucociliary transport. With the cough machine model developed by King et al. [26], it has

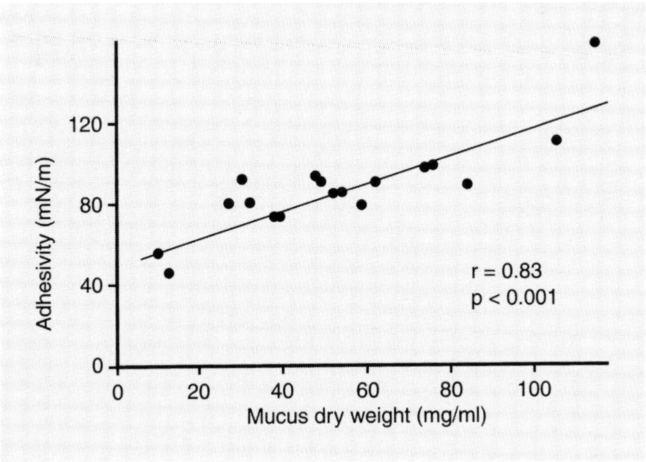


5a

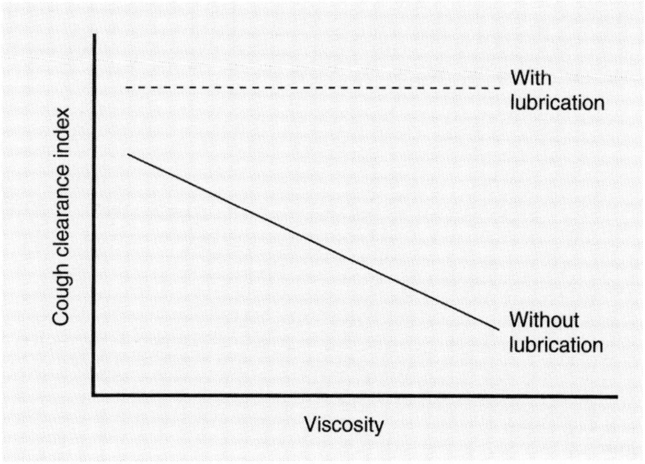


6

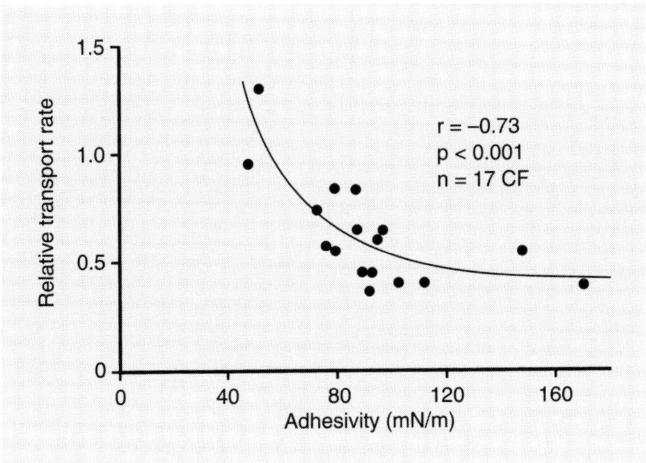


5b

**Fig. 5.** Relationships between water content (expressed as dry weight), adhesivity (**A**) and transportability (**B**) of the respiratory mucus collected in 17 CF patients. The lower the water content, the higher the adhesivity of mucus and the lower its transport capacity by ciliary activity.

**Fig. 6.** Relationship between mucus viscosity and cough clearance index. In the absence of a lubricant layer, cough clearance decreases with an increase in mucus viscosity. Conversely, the presence or addition of a lubricant layer markedly improves the clearance index which does not decrease with increased mucus viscosity.

been demonstrated that the shear-dependent properties of mucus, associated with repetitive coughing, increase the efficiency of mucus clearance [27]. Using a gel mucus simulant to which a sol phase simulant was added, Zahm et al. [28] also demonstrated that in the presence of the sol phase the clearance index was high and did not change with increased viscosity, whereas, in the absence of this sol phase, the cough clearance significantly decreased as the viscosity increased (fig. 6). King et al. [18] suggest that native mucus may exhibit intermediate levels of elasticity as it must be capable of responding to both forms of clearance i.e. mucociliary and cough. Cough clearance decreases with increasing mucus viscosity and elasticity. However, at constant mechanical impedance (ratio of elasticity and viscosity), cough clearance increases as the ratio of viscosity to elasticity decreases. The relationship between cough clearance and spinnability is found to be totally opposite to that which exists between mucociliary clearance and spinnability. This suggests that a balance may naturally exist between elastic and viscous properties of mucus to optimize both forms of clearance. Regarding adhesivity, it has been clearly shown that lowering mucus surface tension or lowering adhesiveness can be beneficial to both mucociliary and cough clearance. As mucus is a shear- and time-dependent fluid, it seems reasonable to hypothesize that coughing, and particularly repetitive coughing, could induce changes in rheologic properties with a parallel alteration in mucus transport [26].

## Therapeutic Intervention

Airway secretions from CF patients are characterized primarily by dehydration, hyperviscoelasticity and increased adhesiveness. Pharmacologic strategies should therefore aim at improving mucus hydration, fluidity and

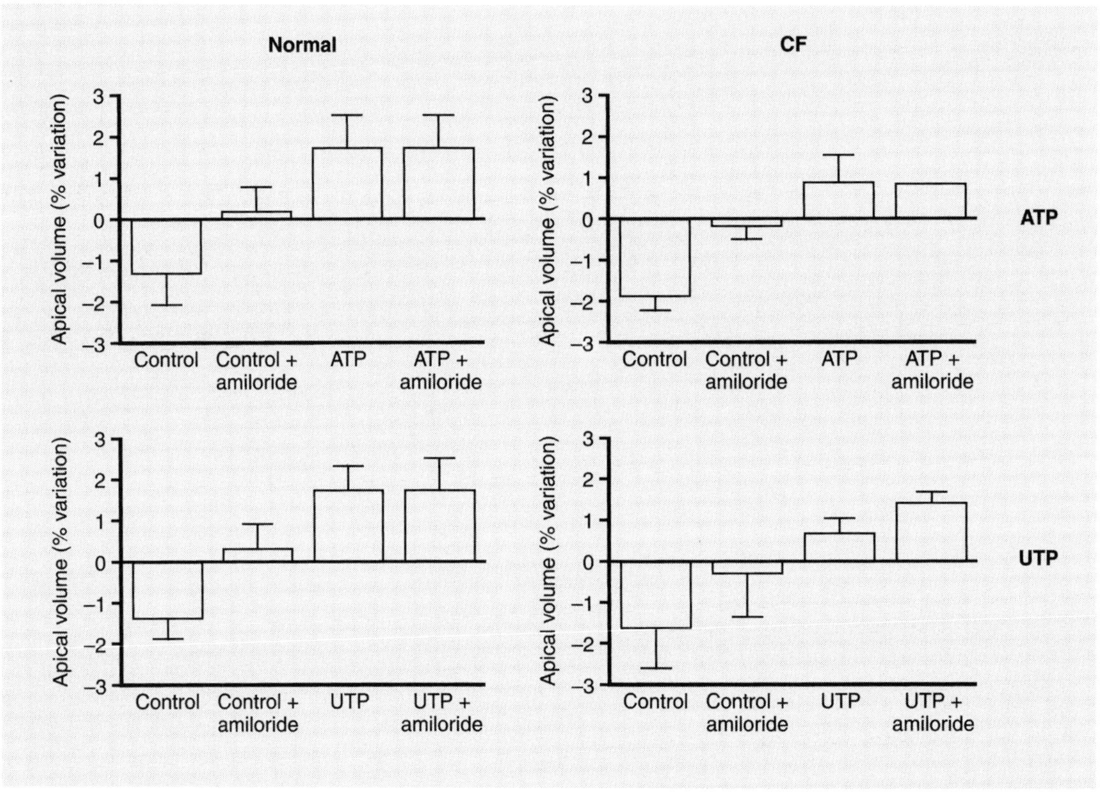


**Fig. 7.** Changes in apical volume have been measured according to the technique developed by Benali et al. [36] after the nasal cells from normal or CF patients have been cultured at confluency on a double compartment chamber. In normal (N) as in cystic fibrosis (CF) nasal epithelium, there is a net absorption under basal conditions (control). Inhibition of water absorption is observed after amiloride incubation in N as in CF. The addition of ATP and UTP, with or without amiloride, at 100 $\mu M$ shifts the properties of nasal culture epithelium from absorptive to secretory.

lubrication and thus restore effective mucociliary transport and cough clearance.

*Hydration*

The CF airway epithelium exhibits two defects in ion transport which are related to abnormal mucus transport; excessive sodium absorption and limited or absent chloride secretion [29]. Both defects contribute to mucus dehydration and, therefore, to the hyperviscosity and hyperadhesivity of the gel mucus, decreased thickness of the periciliary layer, decreased mucociliary transport and decreased mucus and cough clearance.

There is no evidence that oral water intake or inhalation of bland aerosols, which add water directly to airway mucus, is effective in improving the rheologic properties of mucus, increasing ciliary clearance or increasing mucus transport [30]. This is not surprising as the water added to the mucus via aerosol administration is likely to be rapidly bound to HMW glycoproteins (mucins), thus inducing a 'gel swell' rather than providing a layer of water at the gel phase/periciliary layer interface. As ion and water secretion and hydration of mucus is an active process, a positive pharmacologic intervention should aim at restoring a local periciliary water layer by inducing chloride secretion and, at the same time, limiting sodium reabsorption. Knowles et al. [31] have shown that amiloride, applied directly to the luminal side of the respiratory epithelium, is able to 'normalize' the increased transepithelial potential difference in patients with CF.

Acute and long-term amiloride inhalation has also been shown to increase mucociliary and cough clearance in CF patients [32]. Nevertheless, a recent European study [33] has demonstrated that the administration of amiloride, in conjunction with bronchodilators and/or antibiotics, does not result in any demonstrable improvement in lung function compared with placebo.

Recent studies have demonstrated that the extracellular triphosphate nucleotides, ATP and UTP, are highly effective chloride secretagogues when applied to the apical ciliated surface of human airway epithelia in vivo as well as in vitro [34]. This stimulatory activity is thought to be mediated by the activation of calcium transport through epithelial $P_2$ receptors [35]. It can be predicted that nucleotide-induced chloride secretion will increase fluid secretion, resulting in the restoration of a periciliary layer and facilitation of mucus clearance. We have recently demonstrated [36] that ATP or UTP applied to the apical surface of the respiratory epithelial cells, either with or without amiloride pretreatment, result in an improvement in fluid transport which leads to hydration of the epithelial cell surface and reconstitution of the watery periciliary layer. We have also observed that in non-CF, as in CF, the properties of the airway epithelium shift from absorptive to secretory (fig. 7). At the same ATP concentration (100 $\mu M$) as that used for measuring the change in fluid transport, we noted that the nucleotide induced a marked increase in ciliary beating frequency which could be maintained for 2 h (fig. 8).

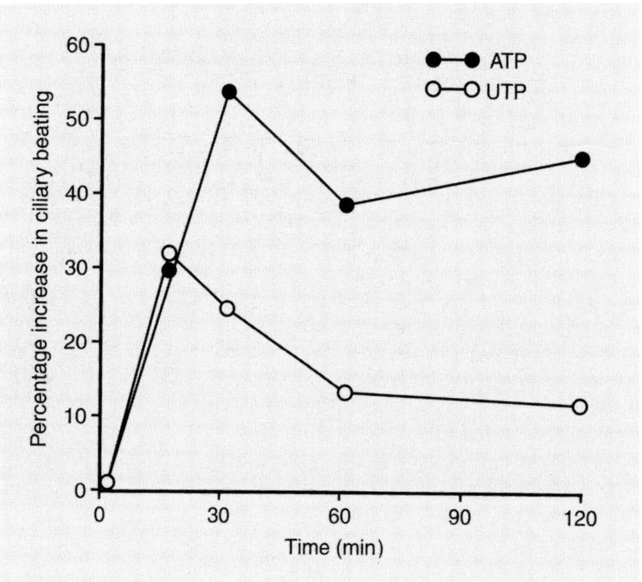


**Fig. 8.** Addition of extracellular nucleotides (ATP or UTP, at 100 $\mu M$) to the outgrowth culture of a CF nasal polyp markedly enhances the ciliary beating frequency of the ciliated cells (30% increase at 15 min for ATP and UTP and up to 55% increase for ATP after 30 min).

The administration of a UTP/amiloride combination has also been demonstrated to improve small airway clearance to near-normal basal rates in a very recent study in CF patients [37].

*Fluidification*

Alternative therapeutic approaches to restoring normal respiratory function in CF involve the application of molecules that are capable of altering the rheologic (hyperviscous) and physical (hyperadhesive) properties of CF mucus. Airway secretions may be fluidified by cleaving those molecules which contribute to its increased viscoelasticity such as DNA. The viscoelastic properties of purulent secretions result primarily from the presence of highly polymerized polyanionic deoxyribonucleic acid (DNA). A highly purified recombinant form of human deoxyribonuclease I (rhDNase) has recently been produced and characterized [38], and has been demonstrated to improve the rheologic properties of CF secretions, with a corresponding reduction in the length of the mucus DNA 'strands'.

In CF patients, inhalation of rhDNase has resulted in improved lung function and reduced respiratory tract infections requiring parenteral antibiotics in the absence of any toxic effects [39]. We have recently demonstrated in vitro that the incubation of rhDNase with CF mucus, which has a low mucociliary and cough transport capacity, induces a significant improvement in mucus clearability and an associated improvement in viscoelasticity (fig. 9). Even at low concentrations (0.2 µg/ml), a significant reduction in viscosity could be demonstrated. We also showed that rhDNase could improve the mucus surface properties [40].

Other agents, still at a pre-phase I stage in their clinical development, may also have therapeutic potential in modifying CF mucus abnormalities. Vasconcellos et al. [41] have recently shown that filamentous actin is present in CF sputum samples and that gelsolin, an agent which cleaves these filaments, is able to reduce sputum viscosity in a dose-dependent manner. The use of combination treatments, such as rhDNase and gene therapy, or even sequential regimens, such as mucolytic drugs prior to gene therapy represent interesting potential future treatment options. Treatment with rhDNase prior to gene therapy could result in more widespread transfection of recombinant CFTR cDNA by obliterating the physical barrier formed by the unusually viscous mucus gel layer.

*Lubrication*

In addition to true 'mucolytic' agents, which act primarily by reducing mucus viscoelasticity, 'surface-active' phospholipids such as phosphatidylglycerol may have therapeutic potential in CF by improving mucus cleara-

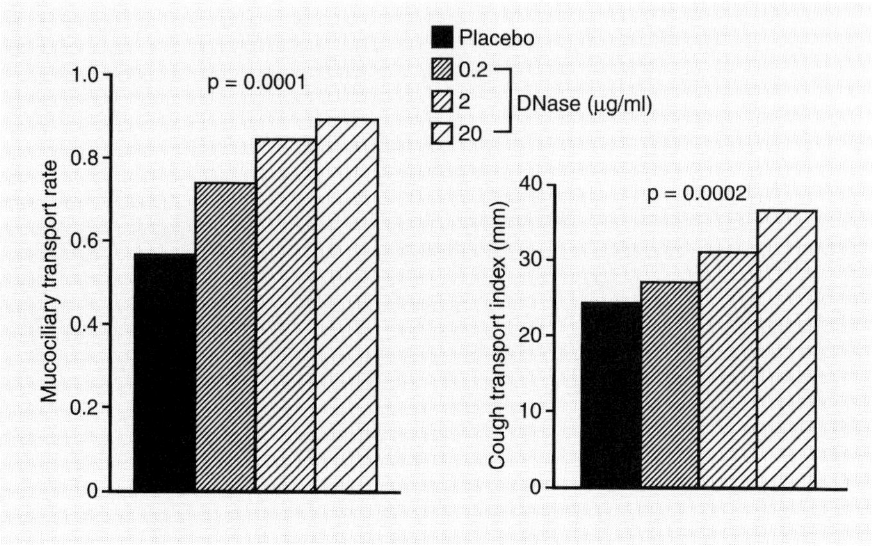


**Fig. 9.** Dose-dependent effect of rhDNase on the transport of CF mucus by ciliary activity (frog palate model) or by cough transport (simulated cough machine). In all the 11 CF mucus samples characterized by an initial low relative mucociliary transport rate (<0.7), rhDNase significantly improves the mucociliary and cough transport rates (p = 0.0001 and p = 0.0002, respectively).

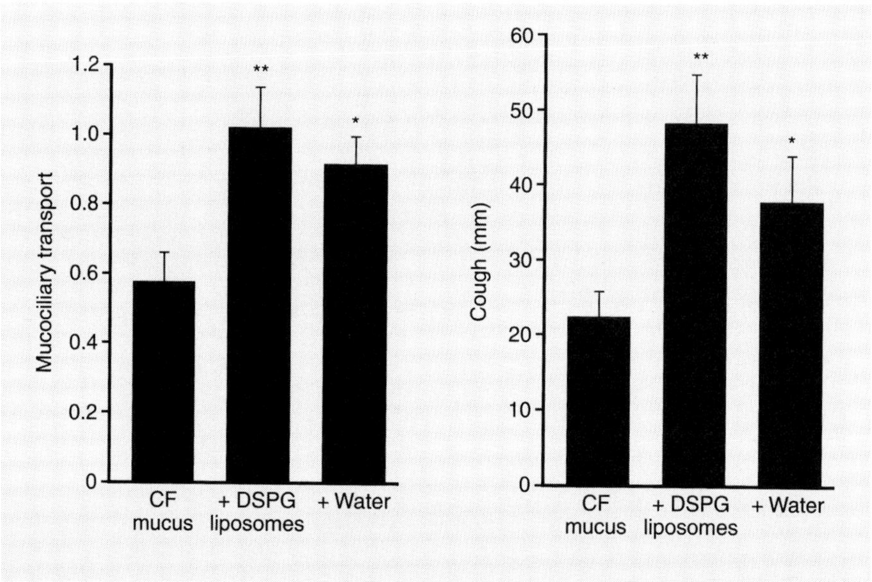


**Fig. 10.** Effects of addition of DSPG liposomes and water to native CF mucus transport by cough or mucociliary mechanisms. * = $p < 0.05$; ** = $p < 0.001$.

bility. Administration of distearoyl phosphatidylglycerol (DSPG) may enable the surface-active phospholipid fraction to be restored [26]. This deficient fraction contributes, together with dehydration, to the marked adhesiveness and stickiness responsible for impairment of mucus transport and severe bronchial obstruction.

Supplementing exogenous surfactant in the trachea has already been proposed for the treatment and prevention of respiratory distress in premature infants. Girod de Bentzmann et al. [42] have shown in vitro that the transport of mucus by ciliary activity and cough may be significantly enhanced by coating the mucus with liposomes of DSPG (fig. 10). These liposomes did not cause any toxicity to the human respiratory surface epithelial cells, suggesting that the administration of liposomes by aerosol or instillation could be a very promising future strategy for the treatment of bronchial obstruction due to hypersecretion. In addition to their potential therapeutic use in patients with hyperviscous and hyperadhesive airway secretions, these liposomes could provide a hydrophobic barrier to deleterious *Pseudomonas aeruginosa* exoproducts. DSPG liposomes have also been demonstrated to decrease *P. aeruginosa* adherence to migrating respiratory cells which mimic regenerating epithelium following injury [43].

## Conclusion

In conclusion, CF airway secretions are characterized by dehydration, increased glycoprotein, protein (either serum-derived or locally synthesized) lipid and DNA content, and related physical and rheologic abnormalities. These abnormalities undoubtedly contribute to inefficient mucus transport, leading to mucus stagnation, bacterial colonization and progressive bronchial obstruction. Therapeutic interventions which aim at restoring efficient mucociliary and cough clearance should focus on the correction of the rheologic and physical mucus abnormalities through rehydration, fluidification and lubrication.


## Acknowledgements

This work was supported by INSERM and by grants from MESR (94 CO 137), Synthelabo (87118) and from the Association Française de Lutte contre la Mucoviscidose (AFLM).


## References


1 Lopez-Vidriero MT, Das I, Smith P, Picot R, Reid L: Bronchial secretion from normal human airways after inhalation of prostaglandins $F_2\alpha$, acetylcholine, histamine and citric acid. Thorax 1977;32:734–739.

2 Matthews LM, Spector S, Lemon J, Potter JL: Studies on pulmonary secretions. Am Rev Respir Dis 1963;88:199–204.

3 Bhaskar KR, O'Sullivan DP, Seltzer J, Rossing TH, Drazen JM, Reid L: Density gradient study of bronchial mucus aspirates from healthy volunteers (smokers and non-smokers) and from patients with tracheostomy. Exp Lung Res 1985;9:289–308.

4 Potter JL, Matthews LW, Spector S, Lemon J: Studies on pulmonary secretions. 2. Osmolality and ionic environment of pulmonary secretions from patients with cystic fibrosis, bronchiectasis and laryngectomy. Am Rev Respir Dis 1967;96:83–87.

5 Boat TF, Cheng PW, Leigh MW: Biochemistry of mucus; in Takishima T, Shimura S (eds): Airway Secretion. Lung Biology in Health and Disease. New York, Dekker, 1994, vol 72, pp 217–282.

6 Joris L, Dab I, Quinton PM: Elemental composition of human airway surface fluid in healthy and diseased airways. Am Rev Respir Dis 1993;148:1633–1637.

7 Lamblin G, Lhermitte M, Klein A, Houdret N, Scharfman A, Ramphal R, Roussel P: The carbohydrate diversity of human respiratory mucins: a protection of the underlying mucosa: Am Rev Respir Dis 1991;14:S19–S24.

8 Sahu S, Lynn WS: Hyaluronic acid in the pulmonary secretions of patients with asthma. Biochem J 1978;173:565–568.

9 Rahmoune H, Lamblin G, Lafitte J, Galabert C, Filliat M, Roussel P: Chondroitin sulfate in sputum from patients with cystic fibrosis and chronic bronchitis. Am J Respir Cell Mol Biol 1991;5:315–320.

10 Girod S, Zahm JM, Plotkowski C, Beck G, Puchelle E: Role of the physicochemical properties of mucus in the protection of the respiratory epithelium. Eur Respir J 1992;5:477–487.

11 Jacquot J, Hayem A, Galabert C: Functions of proteins and lipids in airway secretions. Eur Respir J 1992;5:343–358.

12 Girod S, Fuchey C, Galabert C, Lebonvallet S, Bonnet N, Ploton D, Puchelle E: Identification of phospholipids in secretory granules of human submucosal gland respiratory cells. J Histochem Cytochem 1991;39:193–198.

13 Girod S, Galabert C, Pierrot D, Boissonnade MM, Zahm JM, Baszkin A, Puchelle E: Role of phospholipid lining in respiratory mucus clearance by cough. J Appl Physiol 1991;71:2262–2266.

14 Yeates DB: Mucus rheology; in Crystal RG, West JB (eds): The Lung: Scientific Foundations. New York, Raven Press, 1991, pp 197–203.

15 Puchelle E, Zahm JM, Duvivier: Spinnability of bronchial mucus. Relationship with viscoelasticity and mucus transport properties. Biorheology 1983;20:239–249.

16 Dirksen ER, Sanderson MJ: Regulation of ciliary activity in the mammalian respiratory tract. Biorheology 1990;27:533–545.

17 Liote H, Zahm JM, Pierrot D, Puchelle E: Role of mucus and cilia in nasal mucociliary clearance in healthy subjects. Am Rev Respir Dis 1989;140:132–136.

18 King M, Rubin B: Rheology of airway mucus. Relationship with clearance function; in Takishima T, Shimura S (eds): Airway Secretions. Lung Biology in Health and Disease. New York, Dekker, 1994, vol 72, pp 283–314.

19 Shih CK, Litt M, Khan MA, Wolf DP: Effect of nondialyzable solids concentration and viscoelasticity on ciliary transport of tracheal mucus. Am Rev Respir Dis 1977;115:989–995.

20 Puchelle E, Zahm JM, Quemada D: Rheological properties controlling mucociliary frequency and respiratory mucus transport. Biorheology 1987;24:557–563.

21 Puchelle E, Gaillard D, Ploton D, Hinnrasky J, Fuchey C, Boutterin MC, Jacquot J, Dreyer D, Pavirani A, Dalemans W: Differential localization of the cystic fibrosis transmembrane conductance regulator in normal and cystic fibrosis airway epithelium. Am J Respir Cell Mol Biol 1992;7:458–491.

22 Jacquot J, Puchelle E, Hinnrasky J, Fuchey C, Bettinger C, Spilmont C, Bonnet N, Dieterle A, Dreyer D, Pavirani A, Dalemans W: Localization of the cystic fibrosis transmembrane conductance regulator in airway secretory glands. Eur Respir J 1993;6:169–176.

23 Slomiany A, Murty VLM, Aono M, Snyder CE, Herp A, Slomiany BL: Lipid composition of tracheobronchial secretions from normal individuals and patients with cystic fibrosis. Biochim Biophys Acta 1982;710:106–111.

24 Houdret N, Perini JM, Galabert C, Scharfman A, Humbert P, Lamblin G, Roussel P: The high lipid content of respiratory mucins in cystic fibrosis is related to infection. Biochim Biophys Acta 1986;880:54–61.

25 Girod S, Galabert C, Lecuire A, Zahm JM, Puchelle E: Phospholipid composition and surface-active properties of tracheobronchial secretions from patients with cystic fibrosis and chronic obstructive pulmonary diseases. Pediatr Pulmonol 1992;13:22–27.

26 King M, Brock G, Lundell C: Clearance of mucus by simulated cough. J Appl Physiol 1985;58:1776–1782.

27 Zahm JM, King M, Duvivier C, Pierrot D, Girod S, Puchelle E: Role of simulated repetitive coughing in mucus clearance. Eur Respir J 1991;4:2709–2717.

28 Zahm JM, Pierrot D, Vaquez-Girod S, Duvivier C, King M, Puchelle E: The role of mucus sol phase in clearance by simulated cough. Biorheology 1989;26:747–752.

29 Quinton PM: Cystic fibrosis: A disease in electrolyte transport. FASEB J 1990;4:2709-2717.

30 Wanner A, Rao A: Clinical implications for and effects of bland, mucolytic and antibiotic aerosols. Am Rev Respir Dis 1980;122:79–87.

31 Knowles MR, Church NL, Waltner WE, Yankaskas JR, Gilligan P, King M, Edwards LJ, Helms RW, Boucher RC: A pilot study of aerosolized amiloride for the treatment of lung disease in cystic fibrosis. N Engl J Med 1990;322: 1189–1194.
32 App EM, King M, Hilfesmeder R, Köhler D, Matthys H: Acute and long-term amiloride inhalation in cystic fibrosis lung disease. Am Rev Respir Dis 1990;141:605–612.
33 Graham A, Hasani A, Alton EWFW, Martin GP, Marriott C, Hodson ME, Clarke SW, Geddes DM: No added benefit from nebulized amiloride in patients with cystic fibrosis. Eur Respir J 1993;6:1243–1248.
34 Knowles MR, Clarke LL, Boucher RC: Activation by extracellular nucleotides of chloride secretion in the airway epithelia of patients with cystic fibrosis. N Engl J Med 1991;325: 533–538.
35 Clarke LL, Boucher RC: Chloride secretory response to extracellular ATP in human normal and cystic fibrosis nasal epithelia. Am J Physiol 19;263(Cell Physiol 32):C348–356.
36 Benali R, Pierrot D, Zahm JM, de Bentzmann S, Puchelle E: Effect of extracellular ATP and UTP on fluid transport by human nasal epithelial cells in culture. Am J Respir Cell Mol Biol 1994;10:363–368.
37 Bennett WD, Olivier KN, Zeman KL, Hohnebeker KH, Boucher RC, Knowles MR: Acute effect of aerosolised uridine 5′-triphosphate (UTP + amiloride) on mucociliary clearance in cystic fibrosis. Respir Critical Care Med 1994; 149:A670.
38 Shak S, Capon DJ, Hellmiss R, Marsters SA, Baker CL: Recombinant human DNase reduces the viscosity of cystic fibrosis sputum. Proc Natl Acad Sci USA 1990;87:9188–9192.
39 Ramsey BW, Astley SJ, Aitken ML, Burke W, Colin AA, Dorkin HL, Eisenberg JD, Gibson RL, Harwood I, Schidlow DV, Wilmott RW, Wohl M, Meyerson LJ, Shak S, Fuchs H, Smith A: Efficacy and safety of short-term administration of aerosolized recombinant human deoxyribonuclease in patients with cystic fibrosis. Am Rev Respir Dis 1993;148:145–151.
40 Zahm JM, Girod de Bentzmann S, Deneuville E, Perrot-Minot C, Depret E, Pennaforte E, Roussey M, Puchelle E: Dose-dependent effect of recombinant human DNase on the transport properties of cystic fibrosis human respiratory mucus. Respir Critical Care Med 1994; 149:A67.
41 Vasconcellos CA, Allen PG, Wohl ME, Drazen JM, Janmey PA, Stossel TP: Reduction in viscosity of cystic fibrosis sputum in vitro by gelsolin. Science 1994;263:969–971.
42 Girod de Bentzmann S, Pierrot D, Fuchey C, Zahm JM, Morançais JL, Puchelle E: Distearoyl phosphatidylglycerol liposomes improve surface and transport properties of CF mucus. Eur Respir J 1993;6:1156–1161.
43 Girod de Bentzmann S, Bajolet-Laudinat O, Dupuit F, Pierrot D, Fuchey C, Plotkowski MC, Puchelle E: Protection of respiratory epithelium from *Pseudomonas aeruginosa* adherence by phosphatidylglycerol liposomes. Infect Immun 1994;62:704–708.

Respiration 1995;62(suppl 1):13–18

F. Faurisson[a]
J.F. Dessanges[b]
A. Grimfeld[c]
R. Beaulieu[d]
M.D. Kitzis[e]
G. Peytavin[f]
J.P. Lefebvre[d]
R. Farinotti[f]
A. Sautegeau[g]

# Nebulizer Performance: AFLM Study

[a] INSERM U 13, Paris,
[b] Service des E.F.R., Hôpital Cochin, Paris,
[c] Clinique de l'Asthme, Hôpital Trousseau, Paris,
[d] INERIS, Verneuil en Halatte,
[e] Laboratoire de Microbiologie, Hôpital St-Joseph, Paris,
[f] Pharmacie, Hôpital Bichat, Paris,
[g] Association Française de Lutte contre la Mucoviscidose (AFLM), Paris, France

**Key Words**
Aerosol therapy
Cystic fibrosis
Nebulizer performance
Respiratory disease

**Abstract**
This study was conducted by the AFLM in order to determine the performance characteristics of 12 commercially available nebulizers (6 ultrasonic and 6 jet) used in the treatment of cystic fibrosis (CF). The nebulizers were connected to a circuit which simulated the ventilation of a CF child and CF adult, and were tested using three drug solutions: tobramycin (T), colistin (C), and amiloride (A). Nebulizer performance was evaluated according to the volume of drug solution delivered in 10 min during the simulated inspiratory phase (VI), drug granulometry (G%), drug concentration modification in the nebulizer reservoir (ΔC), and percentage of efficiently aerosolized drug (EA%). The ultrasonic devices delivered a significantly higher VI than the jet nebulizers ($p < 0.0001$) for all three study drugs. Ventilation rate did not influence VI. Regarding granulometry, higher percentages of T and A were found to be contained in droplets ranging from 0.5 to 5.0 μm following ultrasonic nebulization. Drug concentration modifications were independent of the nebulizer used but were influenced by drug type; overconcentrations of T and A were observed (ΔC = +10.5 ± 18.6 and +13.4 ± 8.9%, respectively). On average, the ultrasonic devices achieved a higher EA% than the jet nebulizers (17.3 ± 6.7 and 9.7 ± 9.6%, respectively). This study highlights the significant variability in performance of different nebulizer types and emphasizes the importance of accurately testing nebulizers prior to clinical use so that the most efficacious nebulizer/drug combinations may be prescribed.

## Introduction

Aerosol delivery is becoming an essential mode of administration in the treatment of a variety of respiratory diseases, with marked efficacy proven particularly in the treatment of respiratory infections in cystic fibrosis (CF) patients.

In contrast to other routes of administration, the dose of inhaled drug that actually reaches the target site may be extremely variable. Treatment outcome is therefore dependent upon the amount of drug deposited in the airways, which is in turn influenced by numerous factors, including nebulizer type, drug solution, volume of solution in nebulizer reservoir, respiratory pattern, etc. Un-

Dr. F. Faurisson
INSERM
170, boulevard Ney
F–75877 Paris Cedex 19 (France)


0025–7931/95/0627–0013
$8.00/0

fortunately, very little information is available on nebulizer performance in different therapeutic settings. This makes it extremely difficult to prescribe optimal aerosol therapy, and, as a result, administration has become rather haphazard.

## Study Objective

The Association Française de Lutte contre la Mucoviscidose (AFLM) has conducted a study using a breathing pattern simulator in order to determine the performances of various commercially available nebulizers for the delivery of three drugs used in CF treatment.

## Materials and Methods

*Nebulizers*

A total of 12 nebulizers were tested (with the agreement of their manufacturers): 6 jet nebulizers (ARP 7®, Pierre Médical, France; NL 5®, Diffusion Technique Française, France; NL 7®, Diffusion Technique Française, France; Optineb®, Air Liquide, France; Pari Boy®, Pari, Germany; Respirjet®, Kendall, UK) and 6 ultrasonic nebulizers (DF 31®, AGA, France; DP 100®, DP Médical, France; Laboneb®, Laboélectrofrance, France; Portasonic®, Devilbiss, USA; SAM LS®, SAM, France and NU 52®, Europe Médical, France).

*Drugs*

Three drugs were used: tobramycin (T: Nebcin®, Lilly, France, 75 mg/1.5 ml), colistin (C: Colimycine®, Roger Bellon, France, 1MU–3.33 mg/3 ml) and amiloride (A: Pharmacie centrale des Hôpitaux de Paris, 1.5 mg/5 ml). The volume of dilution of each drug was in accordance with the manufacturers' recommendations for each application.

Nebulizers were connected to a circuit which simulated the ventilation of a CF child ($RV_1$: 250 ml × 25 $min^{-1}$, I/E = ½) and a CF adult ($RV_2$: 350 ml × 20 $min^{-1}$, I/E = ½). The duration of aerosol administration was 10 min; however, only aerosol delivered during the inspiratory phase was considered.

*Determination of Nebulizer Performance*

In each of the 72 simulated clinical settings (12 nebulizers × 3 drugs × 2 ventilatory regimens) the following data were collected:

- Percentage of aerosol mass contained in droplets with diameter ranging from 0.5 to 5 µm (G%), considered as adapted to lung deposition. Granulometry was determined using a laser diffraction method (Malvern Mastersizer II®).
- Volume of solution delivered in 10 min during the inspiratory phase (VI) by weighing the complete (filled) device before ($V_0$) and after nebulization ($V_{10}$) assuming a solution density of 1.0 (Mettler PK 4800 balance). In order to account for the variability of the initial volume of dilution, the delivered volume was expressed as a percentage of the total dose (VI%).
- Drug concentration modification (ΔC) in nebulizer reservoir before ($C_0$) and after nebulization ($C_{10}$), assessed using a microbiologic method for C, an immunologic method (Cobas Mira®) for T and an HPLC method for A. An increase in reservoir drug concentration was taken to reflect a preferential delivery of water than drug, for which the fraction of delivered drug was calculated as:

$$DD\% = [(V_0 \times C_0) - (V_{10} \times C_{10})]/[V_0 \times C_0]$$

A decrease in reservoir drug concentration was considered to indicate a possible progressive degradation of drug during nebulization. In this case, the fraction of delivered drug was calculated as:

$$DD\% = [(V_0 - V_{10}) \times (C_0 + C_{10})/2]/[V_0 \times C_0].$$

- Percentage of efficiently aerosolized (EA%) drug, defined as the fraction of DD% with adapted granulometry: EA% = DD% × G%.

*Statistical Methods*

According to the study design, the influence of the three crossed factors (nebulizer type, drug and ventilation) on the study parameters (G%, VI, ΔC and EA%) were evaluated using analysis of variance (ANOVA, Statview® software). A p value of 0.05 was considered the threshold for statistical significance.

## Results

*Aerosolized Solution*

The volume of solution delivered in 10 min during the inspiratory phase was significantly higher with ultrasonic nebulizers than with jet nebulizers (2.72 ± 0.98 vs. 1.22 ± 0.59 ml, respectively; $p < 0.0001$) (fig. 1). This ratio (approximately 2.0) was observed for all three study drugs; VI of T = 2.06 ± 1.20 ml, VI of C = 1.80 ± 1.02 ml, VI of A = 2.05 ± 1.10 ml.

The type of ventilation did not influence simulated VI: 1.91 ± 1.11 vs. 2.04 ± 1.12 ml, with $RV_1$ and $RV_2$, respectively.

The volumes of dilution recommended by the nebulizer manufacturers varied from 1.5 to 13 ml. Despite a larger average volume of dilution recommended for ultrasonic nebulizers than jet nebulizers (8.19 ± 3.15 vs. 4.94 ± 1.69 ml, respectively) VI% of ultrasonic devices remained higher than that observed with jet nebulizers: VI% = 34.6 ± 9.0% for ultrasonic vs. 27.3 ± 13.0% for jet; $p < 0.007$.

For a given device, values of VI% were generally similar, independent of the drug. However, a wide variation in dilution volume was observed with Optineb which nebulized 45.3% of a 1.5-ml undiluted vial of T but only 15.6% of a 5-ml vial of A (fig. 2).

*Granulometry*

There was generally no difference in granulometry between the different nebulizers, drugs or ventilatory regimens. Nevertheless, a separate analysis showed a higher G% for ultrasonic nebulizers than jet nebulizers for T (67.1 ± 10.7 vs. 55.5 ± 11.5%, respectively; $p < 0.001$) and for A (66.4 ± 9.2% vs. 58.1 ± 15.0%, respectively;

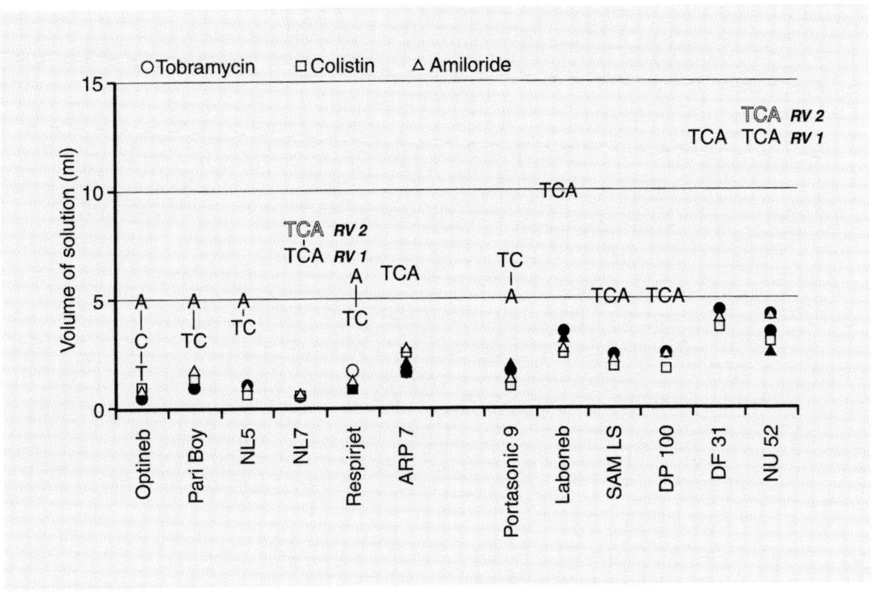


**Fig. 1.** Volume of drug solution delivered during the inspiratory phase for a 10-min nebulization course. Open symbols represent values obtained with $RV_1$; filled symbols are values obtained with $RV_2$. A, C and T indicate the initial volume of nebulizer filling for amiloride, colistin and tobramycin, respectively.

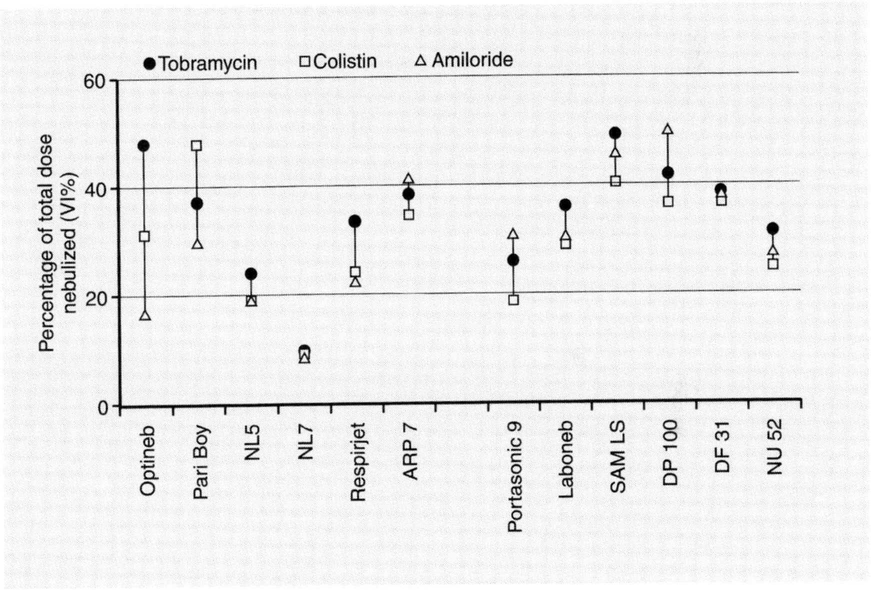


**Fig. 2.** Fraction of drug solution delivered during the inspiratory phase for a 10-min nebulization course expressed as a percentage of the total dose.

$p < 0.05$). There was an inverse, but not statistically significant trend for C (G% = 51.9 ± 22.3% for ultrasonic vs. G% = 55.4 ± 18.2% for jet) (fig. 3). For a given nebulizer there was little variation in granulometry with the different study drugs, except for nebulization of C with DF 31, DP 100 and SAM LS.

*Drug Concentration Modification*

There was a wide variation in drug concentration modification (from –19.1% to +46.5%) with the different drugs, although this was generally independent of nebulizer type (ΔC = +9.9 ± 15.3% for jet vs. +4.2 ± 14.0% for ultrasonic) (fig. 4).

The influence of drug type was highly significant; there was an overconcentration of T and A (ΔC = +10.5 ± 18.6% and ΔC = +13.4 ± 8.9%, respectively) whereas the concentration of C was not modified (ΔC = –2.9 ± 9.4%; $p < 0.0001$ vs. T and A).

*Efficiently Nebulized Drugs*

Therapeutic nebulizer performance was reflected in the results obtained for EA%. On average, EA% was high-

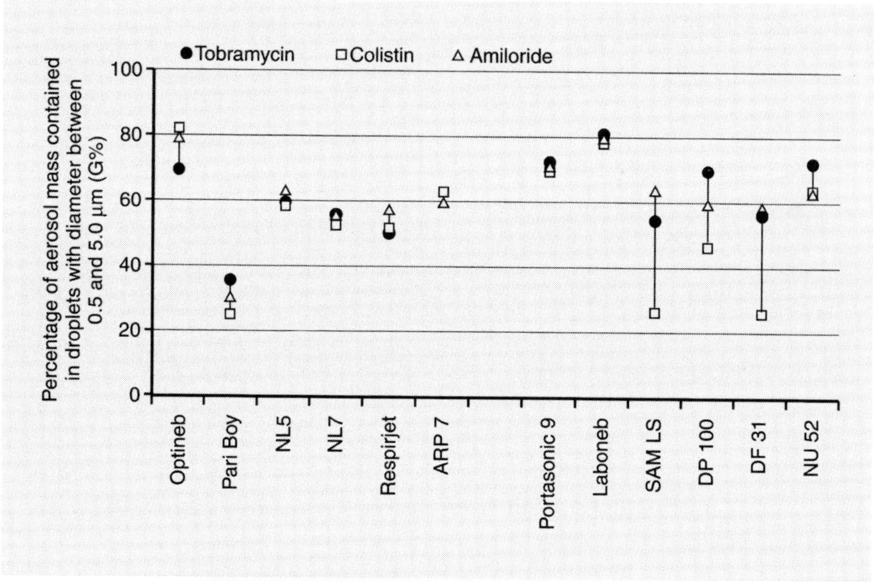


**Fig. 3.** Fraction of mass of aerosol contained in droplets with a diameter ranging from 0.5 to 5 µm.

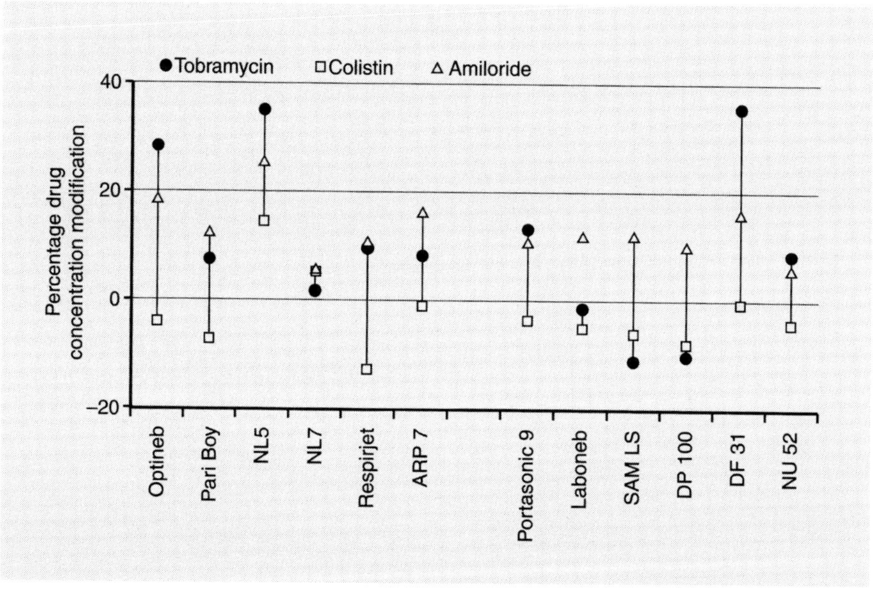


**Fig. 4.** Relative modification of the drug concentration in the reservoir after a 10-min nebulization course.

er for ultrasonic than jet nebulizers (17.3 ± 6.7% and 9.7 ± 9.6%, respectively; $p < 0.001$). However, with C, EA% was approximately 13%, independent of nebulizer type (fig. 5).

## Discussion

This comparative study shows that with a given drug and a given ventilatory regimen different nebulizers have extremely variable performances. From a therapeutic point of view, these differences represent variations in the amount of drug delivered for identical prescriptions which do not indicate the use of a specific nebulizer.

In order to obtain data which could be transferred to the clinical setting, this experimental study simulated, as closely as possible, patient ventilation pattern, considered aerosol delivered in the inspiratory phase only, and limited the aerosol course to 10 min. Simulating patient ventilation reproduces clinical use in CF, as accurately as possible, without the use of additional continuous ventilation. Restriction of aerosol delivery measurements to the

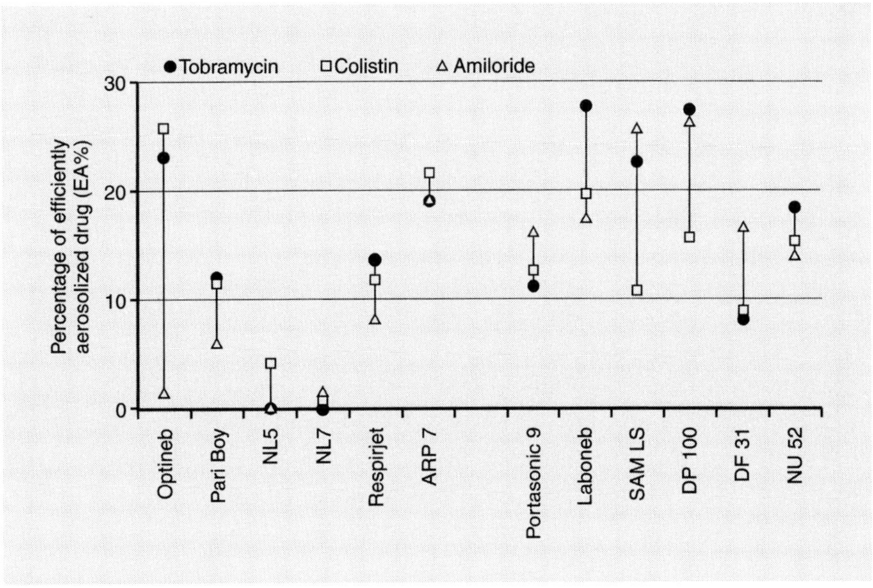


**Fig. 5.** Fraction of the initial dose delivered during the inspiratory phase for a 10-min nebulization course with adapted granulometry.

inspiratory phase is in accordance with efficacy evaluation and allows comparisons to be made between continuous and intermittent nebulization. Limitation of the aerosol course allows an actual comparison to be made between the aerosol flow of different devices because the time to reach the end of nebulization depends on both aerosol flow and dead volume of the reservoir – conflicting variables in the measurement of nebulizer efficacy. Ten minutes was chosen as an acceptable duration of administration as patients have to administer the aerosol three or four times a day.

Granulometry was determined by laser diffraction. Geometric determination of particle diameter is similar to aerodynamic determination when drug particles are in a liquid state, i.e. spheric, and the density of the solution is about 1.0 (our experimental conditions). In addition, the Malvern Mastersizer II® enables particle size to be determined at high resolution (75 channels exponentially ranged from 0.1 to 20 μm). Granulometry was characterized using the percentage of aerosol mass contained in particles ranging from 0.5 to 5 μm, instead of mass median diameter – as this allowed easy transfer to the clinical setting – and geometric deviation (σg).

The values obtained for efficiently aerosolized drug (EA%) were extremely variable between different nebulizers (from about 30% to less than 5% of the initial dose). This diversity has been frequently reported in other studies [1–6]. Efficacy depends on aerosol flow, granulometry and concentration modifications. Therefore, each of these factors must be considered when establishing optimal nebulizer use.

In measuring topography of lung deposition, it is important to ensure that breathing pattern does not significantly modify the amount of drug nebulized. Granulometry, however, does not appear to be a quite important limiting factor; in 80% of cases, the percentage of aerosol ranging from 0.5 to 5 μm in particle diameter represents 50 to 85% of the total mass of drug nebulized.

The lowest values of adapted granulometry are observed in two settings: (1) with the Pari Boy jet nebulizer, independent of the type of drug nebulized; the aerosol particles are of a large diameter and therefore limit its use for bronchial deposition (e.g. for the administration of mucolytics such as recombinant human DNase) [7]; (2) with the ultrasonic devices, DF 31, DP 100 and SAM LS. The aerosol particle size is dramatically higher for C than for the other drugs. This difference may be explained by the high tensio-active properties of C solution. Size distributions of C particles show a simultaneous increase in mass median diameter and σg with multimodal distribution suggesting a coalescence phenomenon following the generation of droplets.

The most frequently observed modification during nebulization was an increase in drug concentration in the nebulizer reservoir. We often observed a preferential delivery of water than drug. This trend was observed for T and A; around +10 to 15% depicts retention of the drug in the device despite an apparent decrease of drug solution in the reservoir. As previously described [5, 6], this important factor, which varies from drug to drug, underlines the importance of testing different drugs when assessing nebulizer function.

The volume of solution nebulized appears to be an important limiting factor when less than one third of the initial dose is inhaled in 10 min. A large variation was observed particularly with the jet nebulizers tested.

Regarding devices with a low aerosol flow, such as Optineb, the volume of the initial dose is an important factor. Such low-flow devices should only be used with low-volume formulations. When the nebulized volume represents only a percentage of the total dose, this volume may be almost drug free in cases where there is a simultaneous increase in the reservoir concentration, as observed with NL5 and NL7.

## Conclusion

In order to adapt prescriptions to nebulizer performance, physicians must have access to comprehensive data appropriate for clinical application. This study indicates that nebulizers should be tested in conditions that simulate, as accurately as possible, clinical use. Different drug/nebulizer combinations have different drug granulometry and are most effective when the drug is contained within a specific volume of solution. If the physician does not indicate the most suitable nebulizer on medical prescriptions, the large differences that are observed in nebulizer efficiency in experimental studies may result into proportional differences in treatment efficacy.

## References


1 Newman SP, Pellow PGD, Clay MM, Clarke SW: Evaluation of jet nebulisers for use with gentamicin solution. Thorax 1985;40:671–676.

2 Huchon G: Effect of different nebulizers on the particle size of aerosolized pentamidine. JAMA 1990;6:33S–35S.

3 Hurley PK, Smye SW: Performance assessment of a range of commercial jet nebulisers; in Technology and Health Care. Amsterdam, Elsevier, 1993.

4 Waldrep JC, Keyhant D, Black M, Knight V: Operating characteristics of 18 different continuous-flow jet nebulizers with beclomethasone dipropionate liposome aerosol. Chest 1994;105:106–110.

5 Dennis JH, Stenton SC, Beach JR, Avery AJ, Walters EH, Hendrick DJ: Jet and ultrasonic nebuliser output: Use of a new method for direct measurement of aerosol output. Thorax 1991;46(2):151–152.

6 Smye SW, Jollie MI, Cunliffe H, Littlewood JM: Measurement and prediction of drug solvent losses by evaporation from a jet nebuliser. Clin Phys Physiol Meas 1992;13:129–134.

7 Cipolla DC, Clark AR, Chan H-K, Gonda I, Shire SJ: Assessment of aerosol delivery systems for recombinant human deoxyribonuclease. Pharm Sci 1994;4(1):50–62.

Respiration 1995;62(suppl 1):19–24

*A.L. Smith*[a]
*B. Ramsey*[b]

[a] University of Missouri-Columbia, Columbia, Mo.,
[b] Children's Hospital and Medical Center, Seattle, Wash., USA

# Aerosol Administration of Antibiotics

**Key Words**
Aerosol therapy
Aminoglycosides
Antibiotics
Cystic fibrosis

**Abstract**
Aerosol administration of antibiotics is an attractive approach to the treatment of the recurrent respiratory infections experienced by patients suffering from cystic fibrosis (CF). Through aerosol administration, drugs can, theoretically, be delivered directly to the target site of infection, i.e. the lumen of the lower respiratory tract, thus enabling smaller doses to be given. This, in turn, should result in reduced costs and decreased potential for systemic toxicity. The efficacy of aerosol antibiotic therapy is, however, influenced by numerous variables, including the type of nebulizer device used to deliver the aerosol, the drug's physical properties, its concentration in the aerosol and particle size, carrier gas and patient factors. The efficacy of aerosol antibiotics in the treatment of CF is controversial. This appears to be due mainly to problems and inconsistencies with clinical trials. However, various antibiotics, including β-lactams, polymyxins and aminoglycosides, have demonstrated clinical benefits when administered by inhalation to CF patients.

## Introduction

Direct application of antibiotics to the airways has been proposed for the treatment of alveolar and bronchial infections almost since their discovery. Indeed, penicillin was first administered by aerosol for the treatment of cystic fibrosis (CF) over 50 years ago.

Aerosol administration is an attractive option as it can, theoretically, deliver the antibiotic directly to the site of infection. This results in the administration of less drug and there is therefore less potential for systemic toxicity. This approach was used for the treatment of pneumonia in 1944 when penicillin G was in short supply [1].

## Aerosolization

An aerosol is defined as a suspension of a liquid or solid particle in a gas – usually air. Various devices are used clinically to produce an aerosol – including jet and ultrasonic nebulizers. With jet nebulizers, the aerosol is produced when a stream of compressed air passes over a small orifice and comes into contact with drug solution. The solution is dispersed into droplets which are subsequently filtered so that only those of an optimal size are inhaled. With ultrasonic devices, high-frequency, oscillating energy is applied to the drug solution, creating sound waves which result in the production of an aerosol as the waves leave the solution.

Dr. A.L. Smith
Department of Molecular Microbiology and Immunology
M653 Medical Science Building
University of Missouri-Columbia
Columbia, MO 65212 (USA)


0025–7931/95/0627–0019
$8.00/0

The output from these different devices is particularly variable when tested with normal saline [2], and there is marked intra- and inter-device variability in nebulizer performance [2, 3]. It is particularly disturbing that there are no rapid self-applied or externally applied diagnostic tests which may be used to verify the accuracy of nebulizer performance.

*Factors Affecting Antibiotic Delivery*

Antibiotic delivery to the lower respiratory tract (LRT) is influenced by a variety of factors, including the drug's physical properties, its concentration in the aerosol, particle size, carrier gas, and patient factors.

The physical properties of a drug have a marked effect on nebulization and therefore influence deposition in the airways. For an antibiotic to be included in the aerosol particle it must be stable under the conditions of nebulization. Because of the large surface area to volume ratio, one predicts that antibiotics susceptible to oxidation would readily be degraded. The antibiotic must also have a minimal effect on surface tension; a low surface tension results in 'foaming' and decreased aerosol production, while a high surface tension prevents the generation of an aerosol as droplets fail to form. Particles with diameters of 1–5 μm are deposited in the LRT [4]. However, deposition is also determined by the extent of sedimentation, impaction and diffusion; diffusion has a greater impact on small particles while sedimentation and impaction affect the deposition of larger particles.

Patient factors affecting deposition include respiratory flow rate (rates greater than one liter per second increase impaction), respiratory frequency, tidal volume, and duration of breath holding (particles with diameters less than 5 μm require up to 2 s to settle in the central and first-generation airways). The specific type of lung disease also affects aerosol delivery. For example, an antibiotic will not reach a consolidated lobe as it is not ventilated.

Overall, the bioavailability of an aerosol (i.e. the percent of the amount of drug initially placed in the nebulizer which reaches the LRT; below the vocal cords), ranges from 2 to 10%. Bioavailability is even lower with certain hand-held jet nebulizers; often more than half of the drug placed in the chamber is not nebulized [5].

## Efficacy of Aerosolized Antibiotics

Aerosol antibiotics have been administered to patients with alveolar disease and bronchial disease for many years. Aerosolization has been used most frequently in patients with CF, both prophylactically and for the treatment of exacerbations, because of the refractory and recurrent nature of their respiratory disease. Efficacy is controversial [6] and is likely to be due to problems and inconsistencies with clinical trials in this patient population. Many investigators assume that their study drug is stable to aerosolization and that the LRT dose is equivalent to the amount placed in the nebulizer. In addition, a number of trials do not have adequate controls: since many of the patients receive an aerosol antibiotic as part of an open trial, or compassionately, subsequent enrollment in a blinded trial may not be valid as they recognize the taste of the antibiotic, and effort-dependent outcomes (pulmonary function tests) have been used. Virtually all antibiotics which are aerosolized have a taste or odor which is seldom masked. In spite of these caveats there is some suggestion that aerosolized aminoglycosides, β-lactams, and certain peptide antibiotics are efficacious in patients with CF.

## Aerosolized β-Lactams

Two crossover trials [7, 8] have studied aerosolized carbenicillin and cephaloradine, respectively, in CF. An improvement in pulmonary function was demonstrated with carbenicillin; however, with the inhaled cephaloradine, no difference was noted in the incidence of respiratory tract infections, hospital admissions, clinical scores, radiographic scores, or the rate of decline in pulmonary function.

## Aerosolized Polymyxin

Antibiotics of the polymyxin class (colistin sulfate, colistinemethate and polymyxin B) have also been administered by aerosol to CF patients. Aerosolized colistin has been studied by Hoiby et al. [9, 10]. In these studies, the peptide antibiotic was administered alone or in conjunction with oral ciprofloxacin [10]. There was a decrease in the rate of deterioration in pulmonary function and in the frequency of *Pseudomonas aeruginosa* recovery from respiratory tract secretions. Since R plasmid-mediated antibiotic resistance to polymyxin has not been described, it is unlikely that there will be emergence of polymyxin-resistant *P. aeruginosa*. However, there may be emergence of other potentially pathogenic bacteria intrinsically resistant to polymyxin (such as *Serratia marcescens,* or *Burkholderia cepacia).* In addition, antibiotics of this class

**Table 1.** Studies of efficacy of aerosolized colistin/polymyxin

| Study | n | Amount[1] units | Design | Duration months | Significant outcome measure |
|---|---|---|---|---|---|
| Littlewood et al. [12] | 7 | 500,000 b.i.d. | open | ? | decrease in clinical score |
| Jensen et al. [9] | 40 | 1,000,000 b.i.d. | saline control | 3 | FVC |
| Valerius et al. [10] | 26 | 1,000,000 b.i.d. | 3-week courses with ciprofloxacin at first *P. aeruginosa* | 27 | less *P. aeruginosa* |

[1] Amount in nebulizer and frequency.

have been reported to cause bronchospasm; aerosol administration of polymyxin has precipitated respiratory failure [11]. This effect is apparently due to polymyxin, as this antibiotic is dispensed without preservatives (see table 1 for summary).

## Aerosolized Aminoglycosides

Aminoglycosides have been administered by aerosol since 1950 [13]. As these agents are poorly absorbed across mucosal surfaces, they are a particularly attractive option for aerosol administration. In most studies of aerosolized aminoglycosides, the aerosol is added to a parenteral regimen consisting of the same aminoglycoside and a β-lactam. Thus, any improvement in pulmonary function is superimposed on that which normally occurs with parenteral therapy [14–16].

In studies of aerosol aminoglycoside therapy alone, both controlled and uncontrolled studies indicate that aerosol administration of tobramycin improves lung function in CF patients [17–21] (table 2). In these studies, other outcome indicators such as antibody titer to certain *P. aeruginosa* exoproducts, incidence of *P. aeruginosa* cultures, and pulmonary function, improved. However, these studies were associated with caveats similar to those mentioned above (the antibiotic aerosol was not characterized, and the dose placed in the nebulizer was generally standard – usually 80 mg, the amount available in a standard 2-ml vial). Although there were no adverse events in any of these studies [17–21], it is of concern that the standard intravenous formulation of tobramycin used contains phenol, EDTA, and sodium bisulfite, agents which could be expected to produce airway irritation. Preservative-free tobramycin, aerosolized at a dose expected to achieve sputum concentrations able to overcome sputum antagonism [22], proved to be efficacious in patients with CF [21]. In this study, drug taste was masked by inclusion of quinine in placebo as well as drug formulations. We found that aerosolized tobramycin decreased sputum bacterial density and improved pulmonary function [21]. The antibiotic was administered at 1-month intervals in a crossover design. No ototoxicity or renal toxicity was observed. This was expected, as administration of the same formulation at the same dose for 3 months to 22 CF patients had not previously resulted in any detectable nephrotoxicity or ototoxicity [20]. Aerosolized aminoglycosides have previously been reported to adversely affect pulmonary function; an acute reduction in $FEV_1$ was reported by Dally et al. [23]. However, it should be noted that the patients in this latter study had reactive airway disease and the observed reduction in $FEV_1$ was also seen with normal saline; the composition of the gentamicin formulation used was not given.

## Antibiotic Resistance

Application of antibiotics to surfaces which contain large numbers of different species of bacteria can select antibiotic-resistant bacteria by two mechanisms: emergence of resistant organisms of the primary species, or overgrowth of a genus intrinsically resistant to the antibiotic administered. Both of these events have occurred in certain clinical settings.

When gentamicin first became available for clinical use, topical application to infected burn wounds resulted in the rapid emergence of gentamicin-resistant *P. aerugi-*

**Table 2.** Studies of efficacy of tobramycin aerosolized by jet nebulizer

| Study | n | Amount[1] mg | Design | Duration months | Significant outcome measure ($p < 0.05$) |
|---|---|---|---|---|---|
| Carswell et al. [19] | 6 | 40 b.i.d. | saline control crossover | 1 | $FEV_1$ |
| Steinkamp et al. [18] | 14 | 80 b.i.d. | open | 20 | clinical score FRC/TLC |
| MacLusky et al. [17] | 27 | 80 t.i.d. | parallel saline control | 32 | clinical score $FEV_1$ slope FVC slope $FEF_{25-75}$ slope |
| Smith et al. [20] | 22 | 600 t.i.d. | open | 3 | $FEV_1$ FVC $FEF_{25-75}$ sputum bacterial density |
| Ramsey et al. [21] | 71 | 666 t.i.d. | taste masked saline control crossover | 1 | $FEV_1$ FVC $FEF_{25-75}$ sputum bacterial density |

[1] Amount in nebulizer and frequency.

*nosa.* This experience markedly diminished enthusiasm for topical (i.e. aerosol) application of antibiotics to the bronchial mucosa of CF patients infected with *P. aeruginosa.* In early open-label studies of aerosol administration of tobramycin to CF patients, *P. aeruginosa* resistance was noted [17, 18]. However, the prevalence was not compared to the rate of emergence of resistant organisms following parenteral antibiotic administration, or that observed following placebo aerosol administration. In placebo-controlled studies of aerosol tobramycin administration, the rate of emergence of tobramycin-resistant bacteria has been demonstrated to be similar in treatment and placebo groups (table 3).

When aerosolized into the airways of patients in an intensive care unit, polymyxin (at 2.5 mg/kg/day) was demonstrated to significantly reduce the rate of colonization with *P. aeruginosa* [24]. Importantly, when administered at the same dose in an 8-week cycle, it reduced the incidence of *P. aeruginosa* pneumonia when compared with a saline control [25]. However, enthusiasm for prophylactic administration waned when routine utilization of this therapy resulted in colonization with intrinsically polymyxin-resistant gram-negative bacilli (*Proteus* species, *Flavobacterium* species, *B. cepacia, X. maltophilia,* and *Serratia* species). Feeley et al. [26] reported fatal pneumonia in 11 seriously ill patients, 10 of whom died whilst receiving polymyxin prophylaxis. In these patients, pneumonia was caused by *B. cepacia* (2), *X. maltophilia* (2), *Proteus* species (3), *Enterococcus fecalis* (1), *Flavobacterium* species (1), and *Serratia* species (1). Only 1 patient developed *P. aeruginosa* pneumonia, which was hematogenously acquired and proved fatal. Thus, aerosolized polymyxin was able to prevent *P. aeruginosa* pneumonia acquired through airway colonization, but resulted in an increased risk of pneumonia from polymyxin-resistant bacteria. Alternating cycles of aerosol polymyxin has, however, been demonstrated to decrease overall mortality due to nosocomial pneumonia [26]. Data available in the literature regarding polymyxin efficacy in CF patients are outlined in table 1.

**Table 3.** Isolation of tobramycin-resistant ($T^R$) bacteria in aerosol tobramycin studies

| Study | n | $T^R$ *P. aeruginosa* | | | Intrinsic $T^R$ bacteria | | |
|---|---|---|---|---|---|---|---|
| | | before T | after T | after P | before T | after T | after P |
| Carswell et al. [19] | 9 | 1 | 2 | 1 | NC | NC | NC |
| Steinkamp et al. [18] | 14 | ND | 5 | ND | NC | NC | NC |
| MacLusky et al. [17] | 27 | 2 | 4 | 0 | 10 | 1 | 3 |
| Smith et al. [20] | 22 | 1 | 2 | ND | 0 | 1 | ND |
| Ramsey et al. [21] | 71[1] | 2 | 2 | 4 | 3 | 3 | 3 |
| | 71[2] | 2 | 2 | 2 | 3 | 4 | 4 |

T = Tobramycin; P = placebo; ND = not done; NC = not commented.
1 After first period.
2 After crossover.

## Conclusion

Antibiotics can be aerosolized to the LRT of patients with pulmonary infections. However, the rational design of an antibiotic aerosol treatment regimen is dependent on the stability of the antibiotic, its ability to be aerosolized, and the particle size of the drug.

The choice of nebulizer depends not only on drug stability, but on practical considerations such as use in the home and cost. In general, ultrasonic devices generate a greater volume of respirable aerosol than jet nebulizers. Of those factors affecting antibiotic delivery to the LRT, patient factors and severity of disease appear to be the most important. This patient effect is not directly amenable to medical intervention, however, it can be controlled through the measurement of antibiotic concentration in respiratory secretions, seeking a target estimated from the best available in vitro data. With attention to these considerations, aerosol antibiotic administration to CF patients can be safe and effective [27].

## References


1 Bryson V, Sansome E, Laskin S: Aerosolization of penicillin solutions. Science 1944;100:33–35.
2 Alvine GF, Rodgers P, Fitzsimmons KM, Ahrens RC: Disposable jet nebulizers. Chest 1992; 101:316–319.
3 Dahlback M, Nerbrink O, Arborelius M, Hansson HC: Output characteristics from three medical nebulizers. J Aerosol Sci 1986;17:564–565.
4 Morrow PE: Aerosol characterization and deposition. Am J Respir Dis 1974;110:88–99.
5 Kradjan WA, Lakshminarayan S: Efficiency of air compressor-driven nebulizers. Chest 1985; 87:512–516.
6 MacLusky I, Levison H, Gold R, McLaughlin FJ: Inhaled antibiotics in cystic fibrosis: Is there a therapeutic effect? J Pediatr 1986;108: 861–865.
7 Hodson ME, Penketh ARL, Batten JC: Aerosol carbenicillin and gentamicin treatment of *Pseudomonas aeruginosa* infection in patients with cystic fibrosis. Lancet 1981;2:1137–1139.
8 Nolan G, McIvor P, Levison H, Fleming PC, Corey M, Gold R: Antibiotic prophylaxis in cystic fibrosis inhaled cephaloradine as an adjunct to oral cloxacillin. J Pediatr 1982;101: 626–630.
9 Jensen T, Pedersen SS, Garne S, Heilmann C, Hoiby N, Koch C: Colistin inhalation therapy in cystic fibrosis patients with chronic *Pseudomonas aeruginosa* lung infections. J Antimicrob Chemother 1987;19:831–838.
10 Valerius NH, Koch C, Hoiby N: Prevention of chronic *Pseudomonas aeruginosa* colonization in cystic fibrosis by early treatment. Lancet 1991;338:725–726.
11 Wilson FE: Acute respiratory failure secondary to polymyxin inhalation. Chest 1981;79:237–239.
12 Littlewood JM, Miller MG, Ghoneim AT, Ramsden CH: Nebulized colomycin for early pseudomonas colonization in cystic fibrosis. Lancet 1985;i:865–867.
13 Prigal SJ, Tchertkoff V, Brooks A: Streptomycin blood levels following inhalation of steam generated aerosols. Dis Chest 1950;17:304–311.
14 Hoff GE, Schiotz PO, Paulsen J: Tobramycin treatment of *Pseudomonas aeruginosa* infections in cystic fibrosis. Scand J Infect Dis 1974; 6:333–337.
15 Stephens D, Garey N, Isles A, Levison H, Gold R: Efficacy of inhaled tobramycin in the treatment of pulmonary exacerbations in children with cystic fibrosis. Pediatr Infect Dis 1983;2: 209–211.

16 Schaad UB, Wedgwood-Krucko J, Suter S, Kraemer R: Efficacy of inhaled amikacin as adjunct to intravenous combination therapy (ceftazidime and amikacin) in cystic fibrosis. J Pediatr 1987;111:599–605.
17 MacLusky I, Gold R, Corey M, Levison H: Long-term effects of inhaled tobramycin in patients with cystic fibrosis colonized with *Pseudomonas aeruginosa.* Pediatr Pulmonol 1989; 7:42–48.
18 Steinkamp G, Tummler B, Gappa M, Albus A, Potel J, Doring G, von der Hardt H: Long-term tobramycin aerosol therapy in cystic fibrosis. Pediatr Pulmonol 1989;6:91–98.
19 Carswell F, Ward C, Cook DA, Speller DCE: A controlled trial of nebulized aminoglycoside and oral flucloxacillin versus placebo in the other patient management of children with cystic fibrosis. Br J Dis Chest 1987;81:356.
20 Smith AL, Ramsey B, Hedges D, Hack B, Williams-Warren J, Weber A, Gore E, Redding G: Safety of aerosol tobramycin administration for 3 months to patients with cystic fibrosis. Pediatr Pulmonol 1989;7:265–271.
21 Ramsey BW, Dorkin HL, Eisenberg JD, Gibson RL, Harwood IR, Kravitz DV, Schidlow R, Wilmott W, Astley SJ, McBurnie MA, Wentz K, Smith AL: Efficacy of aerosolized tobramycin in patients with cystic fibrosis. N Engl J Med 1993;328:1740–1746.
22 Levy JL, Smith AL, Kenny MA, Ramsey B, Schoenknecht FD: Bioactivity of gentamicin in purulent sputum for patients with cystic fibrosis or bronchiectasis: Comparison with activity in serum. J Infect Dis 1983;145:1069–1076.
23 Dally MD, Kurrle S, Webster J, Breslin ABX: The effect of inhaled gentamicin on ventilatory function. Aust N Z J Med 1977;7:98–99.
24 Greenfield S, Teres D, Bushnell LS, Hedley-Whyte J, Feingold DS: Prevention of gram-negative bacillary pneumonia using aerosol polymyxin as prophylaxis. I. Effect on the colonization pattern of the upper respiratory tract of seriously ill patients. J Clin Invest 1973;52: 2935–2940.
25 Klick JM, DuMoulin GC, Hedley-Whyte J, Teres D, Bushnell LS, Feingold DS: Prevention of gram-negative bacillary pneumonia using polymyxin aerosol as prophylaxis. II. Effect on the incidence of pneumonia in seriously ill patients. J Clin Invest 1975;55:514–519.
26 Feeley TW, DuMoulin GC, Hedley-Whyte J, Bushnell LS, Gilbert JP, Feingold DS: Aerosol polymyxin and pneumonia in seriously ill patients. N Engl J Med 1975;293:473–475.
27 Littlewood JM, Smye SW, Cunliffe H: Aerosol antibiotic treatment in patients with cystic fibrosis. Arch Dis Child 1993;68:788–792.

Respiration 1995;62(suppl 1):25–28

*P. Birrer*

Department of Paediatrics, University of Berne, Inselspital, Berne, Switzerland

# Proteases and Antiproteases in Cystic Fibrosis: Pathogenetic Considerations and Therapeutic Strategies

**Key Words**
Antiproteases
Cystic fibrosis
Neutrophil elastase
Proteases
Therapeutic strategies

**Abstract**
The association between abnormal chloride transport, resulting from mutations in the cystic fibrosis transmembrane regulator (CFTR) gene, and the immunologic processes involved in the development of CF lung disease is poorly understood. However, neutrophil-dominated inflammation on the respiratory epithelial surface is a common finding in CF patients and suggests a mechanism for the immunologic abnormalities described in CF. Of particular importance for the pathophysiology of CF are proteases such as neutrophil elastase (NE) which are released from neutrophils in CF airways and cause direct structural damage to respiratory tissue. In healthy individuals, the deleterious effects of excess protease activity in the respiratory system are inhibited by antiproteases such as $\alpha_1$-antitrypsin ($\alpha_1$AT) and secretory leukoprotease inhibitor (SLPI). However, in CF, antiproteases are outnumbered by proteases and this protective mechanism is rendered ineffective. Restoration of this protease/antiprotease balance through antiprotease replacement therapy is currently under clinical investigation and preliminary results are promising.

## Introduction

Cystic fibrosis (CF) is a chronic hereditary disorder caused by mutations of the CF gene [1–3]. It is unknown how and why the consecutive abnormalities in the transport of chloride lead to chronic airway inflammation, mucus impaction, bacterial colonization and infection. However, it is these respiratory complications which lead to lung destruction, the major cause of mortality in CF [4].

Neutrophil-dominated inflammation on the respiratory epithelial surface is a common finding in CF individuals. Neutrophils are attracted to the epithelium by inflammatory mediators such as leukotrienes, complement components and interleukins to defend the respiratory system against invading pathogens and to preserve its integrity. They contain an immense array of potentially dangerous compounds which, in some circumstances, can be harmful to the body [5]. It is the aim of this brief review to focus on neutrophil proteases, particularly neutrophil elastase

Dr. P. Birrer
Department of Paediatrics
University of Berne
Inselspital
CH–3010 Berne (Switzerland)


0025–7931/95/0627–0025
$8.00/0

(NE) – one of the most powerful of these mediators – and on the possible clinical implications of therapeutic use of antiproteases in CF.

## Neutrophil Elastase

Bronchoalveolar lavage (BAL) fluid of CF individuals contains high numbers of neutrophils, which serve as an indicator of inflammation on the respiratory epithelial surface, and active NE, released by activated or degenerating neutrophils. NE is not the only protease of relevance in CF but is probably the most potent with regard to its quantity, broad spectrum specificity and kinetics of proteolysis. NE can directly damage epithelial cells, degrade many extracellular matrix molecules, interfere with local host defense mechanisms and impair airway clearance [6–10]. The chronic inflammatory process which occurs in the lungs of CF patients is initiated very early in life. Our investigations in 27 CF children, aged 1–18 years, demonstrate the presence of neutrophil-dominated inflammation in 25/27 cases, with free NE present in 20/27 [11]. The youngest of these patients was only 1 year of age. This is consistent with the findings of other investigators showing inflammatory processes in the lungs of CF patients only a few months of age [12].

## Antiproteases

Protease control is provided by antiproteases – proteins which inhibit protease activity usually by interacting with their catalytic site. The two major antiproteases occurring naturally in the lung are $\alpha_1$-antitrypsin ($\alpha_1$AT) and secretory leukoprotease inhibitor (SLPI). In healthy individuals an 'antiprotease screen' protects the lung from protease attack, i.e. antiproteases are present in much higher quantity than proteases [13]. However, in CF adults, antiproteases are almost invariably outnumbered by proteases. Seven of our CF children who presented with no free NE on their respiratory epithelial surface also showed markedly reduced antiprotease activity, indicating that many of the antiproteases present are functionally inactivated [11, 13]. There is, therefore, an imbalance between proteases and antiproteases on the respiratory epithelial surface of CF individuals which is potentially amenable to therapy by antiprotease augmentation. This has been investigated using $\alpha_1$AT and SLPI.

*$\alpha_1$AT Augmentation Therapy*

Intravenous augmentation therapy with $\alpha_1$AT shows good suppression of NE activity on the respiratory epithelial surface but only for a short period of time. The antiprotease must also be given frequently and at high doses. This results in high costs and reduces the availability of $\alpha_1$AT. If delivered in sufficient amounts, aerosol augmentation therapy with $\alpha_1$AT is able to suppress NE activity and to restore the impaired killing capacity of the neutrophils [14]. By cleaving complement receptors on neutrophils, NE impairs their ability to kill pseudomonas [7]. Neutrophils incubated with pretreatment BAL obtained from CF patients are unable to kill pseudomonas whereas the killing capacity of neutrophils incubated with posttreatment BAL is preserved [7, 14].

*SLPI Augmentation Therapy*

Intravenous augmentation therapy with SLPI does not appear to be a promising approach as the antiprotease has a small molecular weight and is therefore excreted in urine at high serum levels [15]. Aerosolizing SLPI reduces NE levels and, interestingly IL-8 levels, on the respiratory epithelial surface of CF individuals. However, the restoration of anti-NE activity remains to be demonstrated in CF individuals [16].

NE induces the production of the potent neutrophil chemoattractant interleukin-8 (IL-8) [17]. BAL levels of IL-8 are high in CF patients, even in CF children in whom there is no detectable free NE and low neutrophil numbers [unpubl. data].

## Vicious Cycle

With the above data in mind, a common final pathway – a vicious cycle of inflammation on the respiratory epithelial surface – can be suggested in individuals with CF. Attracted by several stimuli, neutrophils accumulate in CF lungs and release various noxious compounds including NE. NE induces IL-8 production, which also acts as a neutrophil attractant (fig. 1). This may be a key denominator of pseudomonas colonization and lung destruction in CF. Many other factors in addition to IL-8, NE and other proteases play a major role in the pathogenesis of CF lung disease. These include bacterial and viral components, oxidants, cytokines and complement components. This vicious cycle of inflammation should be a major focus for future treatment strategies which may be highly efficacious if applied as vigorously as current antibiotic therapies.

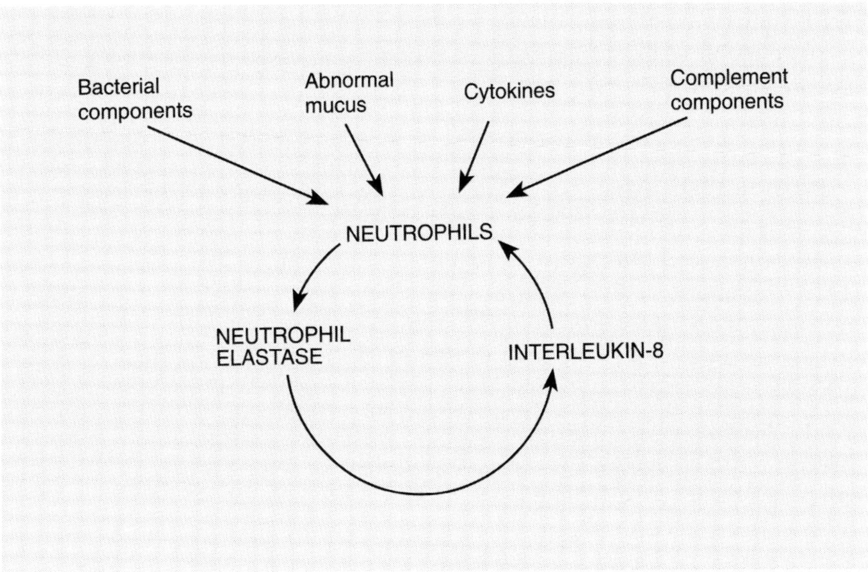


**Fig. 1.** Final common pathway: vicious cycle of neutrophil-dominated inflammation on the respiratory epithelial surface in individuals with CF.

### General Considerations

There are two major approaches to targeting the respiratory epithelial surface: by inhalation and via the blood stream. Both have their specific advantages and disadvantages in terms of crossing barriers and interstitial layers. In CF, inhalation appears to be the most rational approach for many therapeutic agents. Increasing numbers of available drugs make it increasingly difficult to choose treatment which will best suit individual patients' needs, provide the greatest benefits and require little of the patient's time. With evidence of inflammation in the lungs of CF infants, it seems rational to initiate anti-inflammatory therapy as early as possible to prevent lung destruction, and thus increase amenability to optimal therapy for lung disease in the years ahead.

### Future Possibilities

Several years ago, antiproteases were very popular as a novel treatment strategy for CF; many studies were presented at meetings and published in the literature. The limited availability of antiproteases for clinical use and focus on other therapeutic approaches led to a decline in reports concerning these agents. However, the future therapeutic potential of these agents appears to be promising. Although the introduction of antiproteases for clinical use is currently unclear, several antiproteases are being developed, including $\alpha_1$AT (plasma-purified, transgenic, recombinant), SLPI (recombinant) and small molecular weight antiproteases. Several of these compounds are already under clinical investigation, and some will soon be available for clinical use. Biological efficacy has been demonstrated for $\alpha_1$AT and SLPI in short-term studies and a 3-month clinical study with SLPI is under way in Switzerland. However, further clinical evaluation of these substances, and of antiproteases in general, is limited by the short supply of the drugs. Neither clinical efficacy nor feasibility have been demonstrated on a long-term basis for any of these agents.

Antiproteases are a therapeutically promising group of compounds which have an interesting pathophysiologic role in CF and might one day be introduced for routine CF therapy. However, much work remains to be done in this area.

## References


1 Rommens JM, Iannuzzi MC, Kerem B-S, Drumm ML, Melmer G, Dean M, Rozmahel, Cole JL, Kennedy D, Hidaka N, Zsiga M, Buchwald M, Riordan JR, Tsui LC, Collins FS: Identification of the cystic fibrosis gene: Chromosome walking and jumping. Science 1989; 245:1059–1065.

2 Riordan JR, Rommens JM, Kerem B-S, Alon N, Rozmahel R, Grzelczak Z, Zielenski J, Lok S, Plavsic N, Chou JL, Drumm ML, Iannuzzi MC, Collins FS, Tsui LC: Identification of the cystic fibrosis gene: Cloning and characterisation of complementary DNA. Science 1989; 245:1066–1073.

3 Kerem B-S, Rommens JM, Buchanan JA, Markiewicz D, Cox TK, Chakravarti A, Buchwald M, Tsui LC: Identification of the cystic fibrosis gene: Genetic analysis. Science 1989;245: 1073–1080.

4 Boat TF, Welsh MJ, Beaudet AL: Cystic Fibrosis; in Scriver CR, Beaudet AL, Sly WS, Valle D (eds): The metabolic basis of inherited disease. ed 6. New York, McGraw-Hill, 1989, pp 2649–2680.

5 Abramson SL, Malech HL, Gallin J: Neutrophils; in Crystal RG, West JB (eds): The Lung. New York, Scientific Foundations, Raven Press, 1991, pp 553–563.

6 Hubbard R, Brantly M, Crystal RG. Proteases; in Crystal RG, West JB (eds): The Lung. New York, Scientific Foundations, Raven Press, 1991, pp 1763–1774.

7 Berger M, Soerensen RU, Tosi MF, Dearborn DG, Döring G: Complement receptor expression on neutrophils at an inflammatory site, the pseudomonas-infected lung in cystic fibrosis. J Clin Invest 1989;84:1302–1313.

8 Tosi MF, Zakem H, Berger M: Neutrophil elastase cleaves C3bi on opsonized pseudomonas as well as CR1 on neutrophils to create a functionally important opsonin receptor mismatch. J Clin Invest 1990;86:300–308.

9 Fick RB, Naegel GP, Squier S, Wood RE, Gee JBL, Reynolds HY: Proteins of the cystic fibrosis respiratory tract: Fragmented immunoglobulin G opsonic antibody causing defective opsonophagocytosis. J Clin Invest 1984;74:236–248.

10 Hubbard R, Crystal RG: Vulnerability of the lung to proteolytic injury; in Crystal RG, West JB (eds): The Lung. New York, Scientific Foundations, Raven Press, 1991, pp 2059–2072.

11 Birrer P, McElvaney NG, Rüdeberg A, Wirz Sommer C, Liechti-Gallati S, Kraemer R, Hubbard H, Crystal RG: Protease-antiprotease imbalance in the lungs of children with cystic fibrosis. Am J Respir Crit Care Med 1994;150: 207–213.

12 Copenhaver SC, Khan TZ, Wagener JS, Johnson Z, Vasil AI, Carroll NM, Accurso FJ, Vasil ML: Airway inflammation in the absence of detectable *Pseudomonas aeruginosa* by culture and PCR in infants with cystic fibrosis. Pediatr Pulmonol 1994;(suppl 10):A373.

13 Hubbard R, Crystal RG: Antiproteases; in Crystal RG, West JB (eds): The Lung. New York, Scientific Foundations, Raven Press, 1991, pp 1775–1787.

14 McElvaney NG, Hubbard RC, Birrer P, Chernick MS, Caplan DB, Frank MM, Crystal RG: Aerosol $\alpha_1$-antitrypsin treatment for cystic fibrosis. Lancet 1991;337:392–394.

15 Birrer P, McElvaney NG, Gillissen A, Hoyt RF, Leodow DC, Hubbard RC, Crystal RG: Intravenous recombinant secretory leukoprotease inhibitor augments antineutrophil elastase defense. J Appl Physiol 1992;73:317–323.

16 McElvaney NG, Nakamura H, Birrer P, Hebert CA, Wong WL, Alphonso M, Baker JB, Catalano MA, Crystal RG: Modulation of airway inflammation in cystic fibrosis. In vivo suppression of interleukin-8 levels on the respiratory epithelial surface by aerosolization of recombinant secretory leukoprotease inhibitor. J Clin Invest 1992;90:1296–1301.

17 Nakamura H, Yoshimura K, McElvaney NG, Crystal RG: Neutrophil elastase in respiratory epithelial lining fluid of individuals with cystic fibrosis induces interleukin-8 gene expression in a human bronchial epithelial cell line. J Clin Invest 1992;89:1478–1484.

Respiration 1995;62(suppl 1):29–32

*Margaret E. Hodson*

Department of Cystic Fibrosis,
Royal Brompton Hospital,
London, UK

# Clinical Studies of rhDNase in Moderately and Severely Affected Patients with Cystic Fibrosis – An Overview

**Key Words**
Cystic fibrosis
rhDNase

**Abstract**

Clinical data are now available on the use of recombinant human DNase (rhDNase) in the treatment of CF patients with mild, moderate and severe pulmonary disease. Phase I studies were conducted and indicated the initial safety of rhDNase in humans. In the US phase II study, 181 patients with FVC ≥40% were randomly allocated to receive rhDNase 0.6, 2.5, 10 mg, or placebo twice daily for 10 days. All three doses of rhDNase significantly improved $FEV_1$ 10–14% and FVC 10–12% compared to placebo. There was no significant increase in serious intercurrent events but a slight increase in pharyngitis and voice alteration. A phase II study including 71 patients was carried out in the UK. $FEV_1$ improved by 13% from baseline compared to placebo. There was an improvement in CF-related symptoms and no increase in serious adverse events. The phase III double-blind placebo-controlled study included 968 patients with FVC ≥40% predicted. These patients were randomized to 2.5 mg rhDNase, once or twice daily, or placebo for 24 weeks. Compared to placebo, rhDNase-treated patients had a relative risk of protocol-defined respiratory tract infection reduced by 22 and 34% and improved $FEV_1$ compared to baseline by 5.8% ($p < 0.001$) and 5.6% ($p < 0.001$), respectively, compared to placebo. A double-blind, short-term, placebo-controlled study in severely ill patients, FVC < 40% predicted, showed the drug to be safe but there was no significant improvement in lung function. After a further 6-month open-label treatment, patients showed improvement in $FEV_1$ and FVC. Comparative studies using different nebulizers showed that the Marquest Acorn II, Hudson-T Updraft II and the Pari LC give similar results. It appears that rhDNase is a useful new treatment for patients with CF.

## Introduction

Over the last 40 years, median survival of patients with cystic fibrosis (CF) has improved steadily [1, 2], due in the main to ongoing advances in antibiotic treatment, physiotherapy and nutritional management. However, CF remains a disease carrying a significant morbidity and mortality for which new and more effective treatments are undoubtedly necessary.

Chronic respiratory disease is the major cause of morbidity and mortality in CF [3] with progressive respiratory failure due to the accumulation of viscid purulent secretions causing airways obstruction and lung tissue destruction. Experiments performed in the 1950s and

Dr. M. Hodson
Department of Cystic Fibrosis
Royal Brompton Hospital
Sydney Street
London SW3 6NP (UK)


0025–7931/95/0627–0029
$8.00/0

1960s showed that there are high concentrations of DNA in these infected secretions, contributing to greatly increased viscosity [4–6]. It has also been reported that at such concentrations DNA may reduce the efficacy of aminoglycoside antibiotics [7–9].

In line with these early reports, the use of bovine pancreatic DNase was investigated and found to reduce the viscosity of lung secretions in CF [10–13]. However, this approach fell into disuse following reports of an adverse respiratory reaction [14]. The availability of recombinant DNA technology has since made it possible to clone, sequence and express recombinant human DNase I (rhDNase; Dornase alfa pINN) with a primary structure identical to the naturally occurring human enzyme which depolymerizes extracellular DNA. In 1990, Shak et al. [15] provided the first report showing that rhDNase reduces the viscosity of infected CF sputum in vitro. Stable formulations were then developed for aerosol delivery to be used in clinical studies.

## Short-Term Studies

*Mild and Moderately Affected Patients*

A series of phase I studies confirmed the initial safety of aerosolized rhDNase in healthy adults and CF patients [16, 17]. Short-term phase II studies were then performed in the United Kingdom (71 patients) and USA (181 patients) involving patients aged from 7 years, categorized as having mild to moderate CF pulmonary disease (forced vital capacity, FVC $\geq$40% predicted), and considered clinically stable at entry. In both studies, patients were treated with rhDNase or placebo for 10 days with usual concomitant medication maintained. Groups were evenly matched for sex, age, pulmonary function and oxymetry.

In the UK study, rhDNase treatment (2.5 mg rhDNase twice daily) significantly increased pulmonary function as measured by forced expiratory volume in 1 s ($FEV_1$) [18]. Mean $FEV_1$ at day 10 increased by 13.3% ($p < 0.001$) from baseline compared to placebo. Rapid deterioration to baseline occurred within a few days of cessation of therapy. No significant differences in adverse events were observed between the groups and there were no anaphylactic reactions.

The phase II study conducted in the USA produced similar results [19]. CF patients (7–51 years of age) were randomized to rhDNase 0.6, 2.5, 10 mg b.i.d. or placebo. All three doses of rhDNase resulted in statistically significant improvement in pulmonary function: mean FVC increased 10–12% ($p < 0.0001$) and mean $FEV_1$ increased 12–14% ($p < 0.0001$). Again, no anaphylaxis or drug allergy was observed.

Treatment was well tolerated with only a small transient increase in pharyngitis and voice alteration in a few patients.

## Long-Term Studies

*Mild and Moderately Affected Patients*

The main objective of the subsequent 6-month phase III study performed in North America was to determine the efficacy and safety of long-term administration of rhDNase. The double-blind, randomized, placebo-controlled study involved 51 CF centers and enrolled 968 clinically stable CF patients over 5 years of age. Patients were randomized to receive 2.5 mg rhDNase once or twice daily or placebo for 6 months.

Treatment with rhDNase significantly improved pulmonary function. The mean change in $FEV_1$ from baseline was 5.8% ($p < 0.001$) with rhDNase once daily and 5.6% ($p < 0.001$) with twice-daily treatment. Improvement in $FEV_1$ was maintained throughout the period of the study.

Administration of rhDNase was also found to reduce the risk of an exacerbation of respiratory symptoms requiring parenteral antibiotic therapy. Patients receiving rhDNase once daily showed a reduction of 22% ($p = 0.11$) in the need for parenteral antibiotics for protocol-defined respiratory tract infections (associated with four or more prespecified signs of infectious exacerbations) compared with placebo; rhDNase twice daily reduced the usage of antibiotics by 34% ($p = 0.01$). The reduction in risk of an exacerbation was observed in both rhDNase groups throughout the study period.

A series of secondary end-points were also investigated (table 1). Significant reductions were obtained in terms of days in hospital, days on parenteral antibiotics, and days at home due to illness for those patients receiving rhDNase. Treated patients also reported improved perception of dyspnea, overall well-being and CF-related symptoms.

There was no increase in the incidence of adverse and intercurrent events with rhDNase, particularly hemoptysis, pneumothorax or dyspnea. Voice alteration was increased in the rhDNase groups but this was self-limiting and not severe. Again, no anaphylaxis was observed.

Overall, the results of this study indicated that in association with standard care, rhDNase can reduce the risk of exacerbations of infection and improve lung function and well-being in mildly to moderately affected CF patients [20].

**Table 1.** Comparison of rhDNase and placebo for quality of life related end-points (mean ± SE) [adapted from ref. 20]

| Variable | Placebo (n = 325) | rhDNase | |
|---|---|---|---|
| | | once daily (n = 322) | twice daily (n = 321) |
| Dyspnea scale (100-mm scale), change from baseline | 0.4±0.6 | −2.1±0.7* | −0.8±0.7 |
| Overall well-being score (5-point scale), change from baseline | −0.058±0.22 | 0.019±0.024* | −0.004±0.026 |
| Cystic fibrosis-related symptom score (5-point scale), change from baseline | −0.001±0.022 | 0.126±0.025** | 0.112±0.025** |
| Hospital days, mean number | 6.9 | 5.6*** | 5.9**** |
| Parenteral-antibiotic days, mean number | 11.2 | 8.5**** | 9.0**** |
| Days at home due to illness, mean number | 4.8 | 3.3**** | 4.5 |

* $p \leq 0.05$ for the comparison on rhDNase with placebo; ** $p < 0.01$ for the comparison of rhDNase with placebo; *** $p = 0.06$ for the comparison of rhDNase with placebo (Wilcoxon rank-sum test); **** $p < 0.05$ for the comparison of rhDNase with placebo (Wilcoxon rank-sum test).

*Severely Ill Patients*

Studies have also been initiated to determine the efficacy and safety of rhDNase in CF patients categorized as severely ill (FVC <40% predicted). This group represents approximately 7% of the CF population, many of whom are on transplantation waiting lists.

In a short-term, placebo-controlled, multicenter phase II study, 70 severely ill patients were recruited from five centers in the UK, USA and Canada. Patients were randomized to receive either 2.5 mg rhDNase twice daily or placebo for 14 days. Following treatment, improvement was found in both groups for both FVC and $FEV_1$ but there was no statistically significant difference between them. It is possible that hospital admission and intensive regimens of chest physiotherapy contributed to this improvement.

This patient group has been continued on open-label rhDNase for a further 6 months. At the end of this period, clear improvement in pulmonary function was recorded; both $FEV_1$ and FVC showed notable increases above baseline. Mean improvement in percentage predicted $FEV_1$ and FVC was 9.3 and 17.8%, respectively, for all patients participating. No anaphylaxis was reported during follow-up and intercurrent events occurred with no greater frequency than would be expected in these patients [21].

It appears, therefore, that rhDNase is safe and can improve pulmonary function in severely ill CF patients, although it may take a longer period of time before response is achieved. Important data should emerge from a longer-term double-blind study currently being carried out in North America on a group of severely ill patients with CF.

## Administration

It has been important to evaluate which nebulizer systems are most suitable for rhDNase administration. An open-label study has been performed to compare improvement in $FEV_1$ following administration of rhDNase by the Hudson-T Updraft II nebulizer (used in combination with a Pulmo-Aide compressor), the Marquest Acorn II nebulizer (used with a Pulmo-Aide compressor) or the Pari LC nebulizer (used with a Proneb compressor).

The study included 397 mildly to moderately affected CF patients (FVC ≥40% to ≤70%) who were randomized to use one of the above systems over 14 days. Administration of rhDNase improved pulmonary function tests as evidenced by improvements in $FEV_1$ and FVC on both days 8 and 15. No statistically significant differences emerged, with improvements in $FEV_1$ ranging between 12.4 and 14.3% for the three systems (data on file, Genentech, Inc.).

These aerosol delivery systems were selected for this study in the basis of similar in vitro performance characteristics. They appear to provide similar clinical benefit and are currently the systems of choice for the administration of rhDNase. Ultrasonic nebulizers should not be used for rhDNase administration as they may denature the protein.

### Extension Studies

Open-label phase III extension studies have been designed primarily to confirm whether the efficacy and safety of rhDNase treatment are maintained beyond 6 months. Preliminary analysis at 18 months of patients who were originally entered into the key phase III clinical trial indicates that improvement in pulmonary function (approximately 5–6% above baseline) is maintained [21].

Similarly, patients originally entered in the UK phase II study have now been receiving rhDNase for over 21 months and mean improvement in pulmonary function remains approximately 7% above baseline [21].

In terms of safety, rhDNase has been well tolerated in these extended clinical studies with no increase in mortality rate observed in the treatment groups. There are also no significant changes in adverse event profile, including hemoptysis, pneumothorax and dyspnea.

### Conclusions

In conclusion, rhDNase improves pulmonary function and reduces the risk of exacerbations of respiratory tract infection in CF patients over 5 years of age with mild to moderate pulmonary disease (FVC $\geq$40% predicted). Reductions in the rate of hospitalization, antibiotic usage, days absent from work due to illness, and a number of CF-related symptoms have also been obtained. In more severely ill patients, any responses may be less marked in the short term. The results of the current longer-term double-blind trial in a group of such patients are therefore awaited with interest. It has been shown that rhDNase is safe in CF patients with mild, moderate and severe pulmonary disease. The recommended dose is 2.5 mg once daily administered through an appropriate aerosol delivery system.

It appears that DNase is a useful new treatment for patients with CF when employed as an adjunct to conventional treatment.

### References


1 FitzSimmons SC: The changing epidemiology of cystic fibrosis. J Pediatr 1993;122:109.
2 Dodge JA, Morison S, Lewis PA, Coles EC, Geddes D, Russell G, Jackson AD, Bentley B: Cystic fibrosis in the United Kingdom, 1968–1988: Incidence, population and survival. Paediatr Perinatal Epidemiol 1993;7:157–166.
3 Penketh ARL, Wise A, Mears MB, Hodson ME, Batten JC: Cystic fibrosis in adolescents and adults. Thorax 1987;42:526–532.
4 Chernick WS, Barbero GJ: Composition of tracheobronchial secretions in cystic fibrosis of the pancreas and bronchiectasis. Pediatrics 1959;24:739–745.
5 Potter J, Matthews LW, Lemm J, Spector JS: Composition of pulmonary secretions from patients with and without cystic fibrosis. Am J Dis Child 1960;100:493–495.
6 Matthews LW, Spector S, Lemm J, Potter JL: Studies on pulmonary secretions. Am Rev Respir Dis 1963;88:199–204.
7 Potter JL, Matthews LW, Spector S, Lemm J: Complex formation between basic antibiotics and deoxyribonucleic acid in human pulmonary secretions. Pediatrics 1965;36:714–720.
8 Vandaux P, Waldvogel FA: Gentamicin inactivation in purulent exudates: Role of cell lysis. J Infect Dis 1980;142:86–93.
9 Mendelman PM, Smith AL, Levy J, Weber A, Ramsey B, Davis RL: Aminoglycoside penetration inactivation and efficacy in cystic fibrosis sputum. Am Rev Respir Dis 1985;132:761–765.
10 Elmes PC, White JC: Deoxyribonuclease in the treatment of purulent bronchitis. Thorax 1953; 8:295–300.
11 Salomon A, Herschfus JA, Segal MD: Aerosols of pancreatic dornase in bronchopulmonary disease. Ann Allergy 1954;12:71–79.
12 Spier R, Wilebsky E, Pane JR: Aerosolised pancreatic dornase and antibiotics in pulmonary infections. JAMA 1967;178:878–886.
13 Lieberman J: Dornase aerosol effect on sputum viscosity in cases of cystic fibrosis. JAMA 1968;205:312–313.
14 Raskin P: Bronchospasm after inhalation of pancreatic dornase. Am Rev Respir Dis 1968; 98:597–598.
15 Shak S, Capon DJ, Hellmiss R, Masters SA, Baker CL: Recombinant human DNase I reduces the viscosity of cystic fibrosis sputum. Proc Natl Acad Sci USA 1990;87:9188–9192.
16 Aitken ML, Burke W, McDonald G, Villalom M, Shak S, Montgomery AB, Smith AL: Effect of inhaled recombinant human DNase I on pulmonary function in normal and cystic fibrosis patients: phase I study. JAMA 1992;267: 1947–1951.
17 Hubbard RC, McElvaney NF, Birrer P, Shak S, Robinson WWK, Jolley C, Wu M, Chernick MS, Crystal RG: A preliminary study of aerosolized recombinant human deoxyribonuclease I in the treatment of cystic fibrosis. N Engl J Med 1992;326:812–815.
18 Ranasinha C, Assoufi B, Shak S, Christiansen D, Fuchs H, Empey D, Geddes D, Hodson M: Efficacy and safety of short-term administration of aerosolised human DNase I in adults with stable stage cystic fibrosis. Lancet 1993; 342:199–202.
19 Ramsey BW, Astley SJ, Aitken ML, Burke W, Colin AA, Dorkin HL, Eisenberg JD, Gibson RL, Harwood IR, Schidlow DV: Efficacy and safety of short-term administration of aerosolized recombinant human deoxyribonuclease in patients with cystic fibrosis. Am Rev Respir Dis 1993;148:145–151.
20 Fuchs HJ, Borowitz DS, Christiansen DH, Morris EM, Nash ML, Ramsey BW, Rosenstein BJ, Smith AL, Wohl ME: Effect of aerosolized recombinant human DNase on exacerbations of respiratory symptoms and on pulmonary function in patients with cystic fibrosis. N Engl J Med 1994;331:637–642.
21 Hodson M: Data presented to 19th ECFC, Paris, June 1994.